The New Facercise®

Also by Carole Maggio with Mike Gianelli
Facebuilder for Men

The New Facercise®

CAROLE MAGGIO

with Mike Gianelli

PAN BOOKS

First published 2002 by Pan Books
an imprint of Pan Macmillan Publishers Ltd
Pan Macmillan, 20 New Wharf Road, London N1 9RR
Basingstoke and Oxford
Associated companies throughout the world
www.panmacmillan.com

ISBN 0 330 49015 X

Copyright © Carole Maggio Facercise, inc. 2002
Photographs © Ed Ouellette 2002
Carole Maggio Facercise is a registered trademark

The right of Carole Maggio to be identified as the
author of this work has been asserted by her in accordance
with the Copyright, Designs and Patents Act 1988.

All rights reserved. No part of this publication may be
reproduced, stored in or introduced into a retrieval system, or
transmitted, in any form, or by any means (electronic, mechanical,
photocopying, recording or otherwise) without the prior written
permission of the publisher. Any person who does any unauthorized
act in relation to this publication may be liable to criminal
prosecution and civil claims for damages.

9 8 7

A CIP catalogue record for this book is available from
the British Library.

Designed by Roger Hammond

Printed and bound in the UK by Butler and Tanner Ltd,
Frome and London

This book is sold subject to the condition that it shall not,
by way of trade or otherwise, be lent, re-sold, hired out,
or otherwise circulated without the publisher's prior consent
in any form of binding or cover other than that in which
it is published and without a similar condition including this
condition being imposed on the subsequent purchaser.

This book is dedicated to my dear friend Joan, whose inner and outer beauty has, for many years, been my inspiration. To Gina and Jasmina, two young beauties who have helped me stay young at heart and made me realize that you're never too young to start caring about how you look and feel. To Marilyn, whose special inner wisdom has been instrumental in helping me grow and inspire others to be all they can be.

As is prudent with any exercise programme, you may wish to consult your doctor before embarking on the fitness programme presented in this book. Neither the author nor the publisher can accept responsibility for any adverse effects resulting from the misuse of information contained in this publication.

Contents

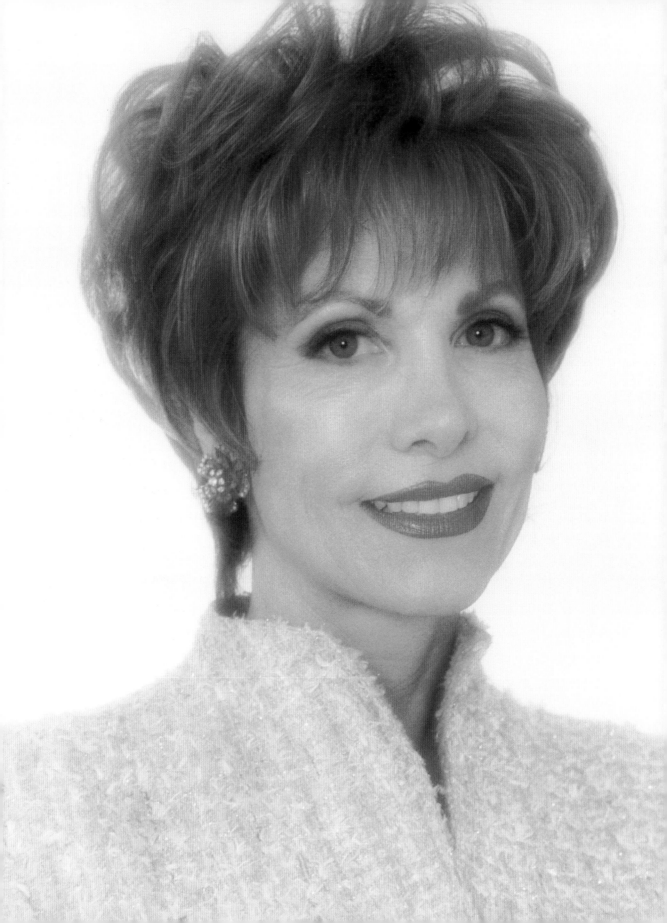

Introduction

ALL BEAUTIFUL WOMEN have one thing in common. It isn't flawless skin or refined bone structure. It is simply that they care enough to make the most of what they have. As the writer Karl Kraus once said, 'Some women are not beautiful – they only look as though they are.' Some people start out with lots to work with while others have to try harder because they have less. It isn't fair, but that's life. To quote Johnny Carson, 'If life were fair, Elvis would be alive and all the impersonators would be dead.'

There aren't many things we can truly control but we *can* control how we look and feel if we are willing to put in the effort. Facercise is your key to looking and feeling good. It unlocks the door to a more appealing facial appearance and consequently a better feeling about yourself. Everyone needs to remember that quality of life depends on vibrant good health and a youthful outlook. Looking young is an integral part of enjoying life. And since the medical community is working long and hard to extend the life expectancy of human beings, why not make the most of the extra years that we can all reasonably expect? We're being told now that scientists think they can extend the human life span to at least a hundred years or more. Woody Allen said that you can live to be a hundred, if you give up all the things that make you want to live to a hundred. That's clever. I would add that if we live anything like that long, we need to look as good as we

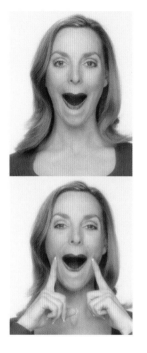

can. Who wants to grow old looking saggy and wrinkly? Who doesn't want to grow old looking good?

I have successfully taught Facercise since 1983 to hundreds of thousands of clients throughout the world. As I was developing the exercises you are about to learn, I consulted plastic surgeons, dermatologists and physiotherapists throughout the world to ensure their safety and effectiveness. Facercise will allow you to recapture and maintain the youthful facial appearance you deserve. By carefully and consistently adhering to the Facercise programme, you will be able to tone and strengthen the facial muscles so that your face becomes more sculptured and younger-looking. With Facercise, you can erase years and lines off your face, without Botox, collagen, surgery or laser treatment.

As you follow the programme, you'll learn to exercise your facial muscles just as you would learn to exercise other muscles with a personal trainer in a gym. A bodybuilder develops certain muscles in his or her body by isolating those muscles and consistently working them. Can the same regime work for the face? Absolutely. A particular facial feature can be developed using the same principle. Because the facial muscles are small and easily isolated, truly dramatic results can be achieved in a very short time span. Just be sure you don't adopt Toni Anderson's adage. 'My philosophy on exercising – no pain, no pain.' Well, we all know we don't get something for nothing, don't we? We've got to travel that extra mile to get what we want. We also know that there's not much traffic on that extra mile. That's good for us if we're motivated. There's no traffic to impede our progress.

Youthful new you

Louisa May Alcott once said, 'love is a great beautifier'. I sure wouldn't argue with that, but I would add, 'so are facial exercises'. Facercise provides long-term benefits and results which are neither costly nor painful. The programme gives you control of your facial appearance and a youthful lift without the expense, the scars, the pain and the recovery time of surgical procedures. In reality, you're your own surgeon, operating on yourself every day, fine-tuning your face little by little, all the time. That's why Facercise, unlike surgery, is not a one-off monumental event, but an ongoing, continuous, step-by-step restoration project.

There are some people out there who really don't like to exercise, for example, American educator Robert Hutchins, who is credited with saying, 'Whenever I feel like exercising, I lie down until the feeling passes.' He was trying to be funny, no doubt. But I am an optimist and my Facercise exercises are suitable for everyone – you can practise virtually all of them even while lying down, so just do it. No excuses. Above all, just be patient. Rome wasn't built in a day. If you practise the exercises as instructed, you will see improvements to your appearance, weekly, monthly, yearly, indefinitely. You will be thrilled with the response the 'youthful new you' evokes. In short, this book can change your life – I promise you that.

Shape your face

MY LIFELONG INTEREST in beauty had a rather unusual start. I was standing in a lift with my mother when a strange-looking lady stepped in. Her face had an unnaturally tight and distorted appearance. I couldn't take my eyes off her countenance. When we came out of the lift, I said to my mother, 'Did you see that woman's face? What happened to her?' My mother said, 'She's had a facelift, Carole. They call it plastic surgery but hers didn't turn out all that well.' I remember thinking to myself that it looked more like deforming surgery, and made up my mind, then and there, that I never, ever wanted to look like that.

I have always felt that looking good makes you feel good, and that it definitely adds to the quality of your life. However, looking good isn't as easy as it sounds. We have to contend with the environment, the sun's rays which can age us, the foods we eat and our non-genetic foster parents, Mother Nature and Father Time. We also have to come to grips with some very daunting statistics: in a recent survey, ninety-five per cent of adults stated that they rely heavily on facial appearances in evaluating another person, and an overwhelming majority of men surveyed said they would prefer to have a partner who had a youthful face rather than a youthful body. Given society's ongoing obsession with beauty, those statistics should surprise no one. But you would think, for a society that puts beauty on such a tall pedestal, that taking care of one's face would be first on everyone's list of priorities, but it isn't.

The good news is that looking good can be made easier with a few simple measures. We just need to pay attention to what we do and how we do it. And we need to exercise. Our ancestors got a lot of exercise simply because life was harder in those days and physical activity was a necessity, not an option. We live longer now because our lives aren't as hard physically, but many, many people do not take care of themselves and they especially don't take care of their faces.

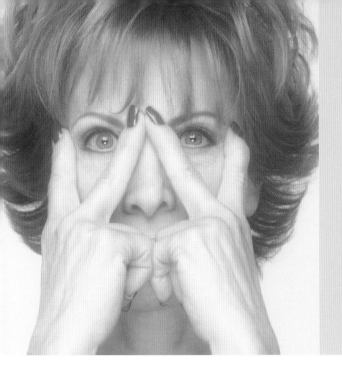

Fascination with beauty

It's been said that there are many roads to beauty. I know I've always been concerned with my looks and I've always been fascinated by other women's looks because there are so many unique and interesting variations. There is a definite difference in a woman's demeanour when she knows she's looking her best. As they say in California, 'she knows she's got game'. My interest in beauty grew while I was in college. I was living in a campus dormitory and some of the girls on my floor would come into my dorm room and ask me to help them with their hair and make-up. We would experiment with hairstyles, make-up and clothes and I was amazed at the difference these changes made in the girls, both in their appearances and in their confidence levels as they left for their Friday and Saturday night dates. It was a very exciting experience for me to see these transformed young ladies. It gave me an exuberant feeling. I knew they could feel it, too.

After college, I married, started a family and initiated a successful career as an estate agent but my mind never really wandered far from the beauty field. I still noticed women's faces, and mentally would make changes to improve on what God had given them. In my mind, I felt my changes really enhanced their appearances and this led me to do some research which became more and more extensive. In my spare time I would read everything I could find in beauty magazines, medical books and journals. I started calling prominent physicians all over the world, who seemed to be on the cutting edge (a pun) of the latest beauty techniques, to ask them questions about the procedures they were performing. The more I researched, the more voluminous my files became. I started to feel like an authority on the subject and this opened the door to a much larger career. I took classes necessary to become a licensed aesthetician and, after graduating, I immediately switched careers, said goodbye to selling property and opened a skincare clinic in Monterey, California, in 1981. At that time I was personally engaged in fierce combat with two of a woman's worst adversaries: ageing and fine lined skin — the results of countless hours I had spent as a young girl baking myself to look beautiful in the scorching Arizona sun. I knew that if I was hounded by these problems, other women were also.

My clinic was a tremendous success and it gave me loads of valuable experience working with many different women. I learned to see how a woman's face becomes a veritable map of her habits, her emotional history and her state of mind. Her face actually becomes an open book to the trained eye. I was able to teach women how to enhance their own unique beauty. I remember occasionally looking into a mirror and, for a split second, seeing a vision of my own mother. She looked tense, stern and tired. Her mouth was pursed and tight under stress. She looked as though she was carrying the weight of the world on her shoulders, which she was. I felt if I could relax the emotional history etched on my face, I could remould and soften my facial appearance. I knew that if I could do this for myself, I could teach others to do it too.

During the time I ran my salon, I put into practice every beauty secret I had. I also scoured the literature and read continuously to glean information on other, newer secrets so that I could pass these useful tips on to my clients. I had capable people running my salon which allowed me the freedom to travel to many different countries to work and study with beauty professionals and to expand my knowledge of the latest, most advanced anti-ageing techniques. I learned to perform anti-ageing lymphatic drainage, which reduces puffiness under the eyes and jawline, and I studied with Dr Gerald Snyder, learning his technique of hand-lift massage (a hand massage which temporarily lifts the face). This type of massage tones the skin and increases the blood supply so rapidly that the recipient looks as though she has just had a face-lift. Unfortunately, the effects of such a treatment are short lived.

I had numerous facial toning machines at my clinic, but they could only bring about limited improvements for my clients. The machines couldn't shorten a nose, enhance lips or widen a narrow, gaunt face. They were tedious to use and my clients had to come back frequently for results, which was costly and inconvenient for them. However, overall, I was extremely busy, my clients looked wonderful and were happy, and I was thrilled to be able to produce such positive results for my clientele.

Discovering Facercise

All was not as amicable on the home front, however. When I was thirty-six, my husband (now an ex-husband), sixteen years my senior, casually mentioned that the fine lines on my face were starting to make me look older than my years. After quickly stifling my initial response, I began reflecting on his comment. It hurt, but instinctively I knew what he said was true. The treatments I was giving in my clinic were not techniques you could perform on yourself at home – indeed none of my clinic employees could do them as well as I could because the techniques were so specialized. I started experimenting with different skincare methods on myself, but nothing I tried could fill in those lines. I realized then that I needed to come up with something unique and different. Something new. Being a licensed aesthetician I was aware that the face contained fifty-seven different muscles. I decided that I had to develop a technique that would build and define the underlying structure of the face in much the same way as sit-ups build and define the underlying structure of the abdomen. This technique would smooth out the lines, tighten the skin and act as a facelift – but without the knife or anaesthetic. Gain without the pain, in other words.

I knew that exercises develop muscles. I researched and studied textbooks, articles and any other information I could find on facial exercises. I discovered, among other things, that, as we age, our faces naturally lose some fat. This fat loss causes the face to take on a gaunt, angular, brittle look. I reasoned that if I could build up my facial muscles, even though I couldn't stop the gradual fat erosion, I could at least achieve the appearance of a softer, younger and even wider face. This I deemed necessary because my face, by this time, was gaunt and getting more so by the day. I began to

study the anatomy of the face and familiarized myself with the functions of the muscles. I read textbooks on the theory of exercise and I studied and experimented on myself until I knew how to isolate and manipulate the major muscles of my face. Slowly and carefully, I began to develop an exercise regime that I hoped would soften the contours of my face, smooth out my fine lines, widen my thin face and open up my eyes.

I was practising what I was learning but I purposely didn't mention my personal experiment to anyone, not even to my clinic staff. I was really just trying to find a way to help me look better. However, one of my regular skincare clients approached me one day and asked me what I was doing to look so much younger. I was taken aback by the comment because I had not noticed any great change in myself. (This is normal. When you see yourself every day, you don't notice many changes.) She said to me, 'Your skin looks so much more peachy and your eyes seem more open and blue.' I told her that I had been developing a facial exercise programme to improve my facial appearance in the same way as I was exercising the muscles of my body with my personal trainer. My client said that she was amazed at the changes I had achieved in such a short period of time and pleaded with me to share my secrets with her. I told her I had not developed a formal training programme and I wasn't even sure if what had been working for me would work for her. I decided that I would like to give her face a try, as an experiment

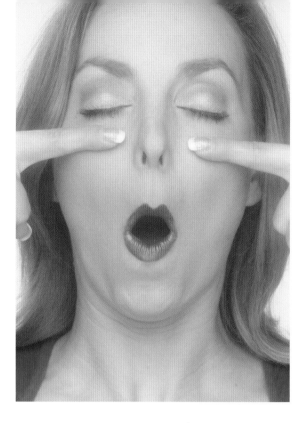

if nothing else. I developed a twenty-two-minute daily programme for her over a five-day period. On the sixth day, I took a Polaroid snapshot of her and the following day she brought in a photo of herself, taken three years earlier. We compared the differences in the photos and we both were shocked. Her eyebrows had lifted, giving her eyes a more open appearance, her cheeks had become higher, fuller and more prominent, her rather wide face had narrowed and her upper lip lines had smoothed out. Her chin and neck were more toned and the soft skin under her neck had visibly tightened. She looked years younger. I was absolutely elated and so was she. In just a few short days, she had learned the techniques to give herself a lifelong more youthful look. I felt, on that day, that the early Spanish explorer Ponce de Leon and I had something in common. He had searched Florida high and low for the Fountain of Youth without finding it. I felt that I had.

My client was so effusive in her accolades for me. She said she would continue to do these exercises for life. I was touched and told her so. I also mentioned that she, not I, had achieved the results. I showed her what to do, but she did the exercises and that is what made the difference. This is something that I continue to stress to my clients to this day. The exercises definitely work, but you have to make the effort to do them. I illustrate this with a cute joke I heard years ago. A down-and-out prays to God to help him win the lottery. He prays and prays and pleads with the

Heavenly Father for the winning ticket. Finally, a voice booms out from the heavens above, saying, 'I want to help. Buy a ticket.' In other words, you have to play your part (buy the ticket). You have to do the exercises if you want them to work for you.

Word of my facial exercise successes spread quickly. After working with many more clients of all ages, I acquired an extensive knowledge of how different faces age. I learned how they could be revitalized, toned and firmed by working the facial muscles. I started giving seminars and classes throughout the United States, working on people with different types of skin and shapes of faces, and with problems such as Bell's palsy, temporomandibular joint syndrome (TMJS) and other facial irregularities caused by genetics, disease and accidents. I showed people how to raise their eyebrows, enlarge the eye sockets, shorten their noses, enlarge their lips and smooth out upper lip lines, make the cheeks appear larger and fuller, narrow a wide face, widen a thin face and tone and tighten the chin, neck and jawline. By now, I realized that every face, regardless of age, shape or texture, could derive anti-ageing benefits from a personalized facial exercise programme and thus Facercise was born. As word spread about the success of my techniques, I expanded my travels and started giving seminars in Central and South America, the Middle East, Europe and Asia. I currently have millions of clients throughout the world who practise my techniques and look younger than their years.

Cosmetic surgery

As my business expanded, I began to research the benefits and drawbacks of cosmetic surgery. I have seen thousands of clients who have undergone plastic surgery with both positive and negative results. Successful cosmetic surgery can rejuvenate the appearance and improve self-image and confidence. But it may not be the answer for everyone. As a person grows older, the bone, muscle and fat under the facial skin actually diminish while, at the same time, the skin starts to lose its elasticity and begins to detach from the underlying facial tissue. It's a nature-induced double whammy. Although surgery can pull the skin tight across the face, the elements that caused the wrinkles and sags are still inexorably at work and, in time, will result in the same wrinkles and sags, which

were evident before the surgery, starting to reappear. The average facelift is estimated to last between five and seven years, so it's definitely not a permanent fix.

Many people, once they get on the cosmetic surgery merry-go-round, find themselves unable to get off. A facelift can sometimes actually emphasize the ageing, brittle look of one's features. I'm talking about the same artificially tight look that I first saw on the lady in the lift when I was fourteen. That vision has been seared indelibly in my mind and will remain there for ever. You've probably had the same experience yourselves. Take a good look at some of your favourite television and movie stars as they start to age. They're riding the cosmetic surgery merry-go-round. Instead of dealing with the causes of facial ageing, cosmetic surgery tends to address the symptoms or results of facial ageing. Facercise works because it deals with the causes of ageing, not the symptoms, resulting in natural, long-term results.

I know that there are cosmetic surgeons who are creative at what they do. But, like Paul Goodman once said, 'many are creative, but few are artists'. If you want a good plastic surgery result, you need to locate a surgeon who is creative *and* an artist. To locate a good one involves a lot of time, energy and research. You can't do too much legwork here. It's your face with which you're dealing so you need to be thorough. Start with referrals from satisfied patients. Interview the surgeons you've put on your lists. Ask to see 'before' and 'after' pictures of clients on whom the surgeons have operated, keeping in mind that no surgeon is going to show you the results of operations that did not turn out satisfactorily. You're really only going to see the success stories. Also remember that not everyone is a candidate for cosmetic surgery. Your health may not permit it. Your skin pigmentation may not be satisfactory and your age may be a factor, too. And above all, don't forget it is possible to achieve results similar to successful cosmetic surgery without experiencing the trauma, risk, expense and inconvenience of going under the knife. You need to assess your options carefully (and your pain and financial thresholds, too).

There are many enlightened doctors who are aware of important adjuncts to cosmetic surgery, such as customized skincare and facial exercises. Many cosmetic surgeons refer their patients to me because they know that Facercise can help reshape muscles weakened from atrophy, accidents, facelifts and other surgical modifications. Dr Lawrence Birnbaum, a well-known Beverly Hills plastic surgeon, in a letter to me, stated that 'in my instructions to patients, I frequently encourage them to do facial exercises'. More than sixty per cent of my clients are people who have had elective cosmetic surgery of some type or another. They've undergone a blepharoplasty (eyelift), a rhinoplasty (nose job) or a complete facelift.

According to statistics kept on the top five cosmetic surgery procedures, the eyelift is number three on the cosmetic hit parade. Facelifts are right below the eyelifts, weighing in at number four, while the number one procedure, at the time of writing, is liposuction. None of these procedures is cheap, either. The average fee for eyelid surgery for both upper and lower eyelids is $3000 (£2400). The average fee for a facelift (not including the eyelids) is $5500 (£3740), which does not include the anaesthetic or other related expenses. As for the costs for liposuction, the average price is around $1900 (£1292) per site and most people have more than a few sites for the surgeon and his cannula to visit. These prices give a new meaning to the word 'ouch'. Not all plastic surgery is successful either and I can sympathize with those people who are disappointed with the outcome of their operations. I had a botched nose job when I was twenty-two that left a dent on one side of my nose and left the tip of my nose appearing too long. I had spent good money for the procedure, gone through some pain and time recovering and I was left with a nose that I felt was less attractive than when I underwent the procedure. I have to admit that I cried more than a few times about how my operation turned out. The Facercise exercises, however, helped to shorten my nose tip and also filled out the dent over the course of several months. Often, when a person has a nose job, it doesn't look as if it belongs on that person's face. Somehow it stands out, not appearing to fit the face. But with facial exercise and increased circulation, the nose can start to appear more symmetrical and natural to the face.

Many of my clients who have had cosmetic surgery are determined not to go back for seconds. They don't want another ride on the cosmetic surgery merry-go-round. In the first year after any cosmetic surgery, I teach my clients to exercise and build up their facial muscles to prevent the need for subsequent costly, painful maintenance operations. Facercise is a quick and inexpensive tool to help control the ageing process. It's painless and there's no down time. No merry-go-round here.

While I am not opposed to cosmetic surgery, it's very important to note that there is always an element of risk (medical and psychological) attached to such procedures. Even the best cosmetic surgeons in the world cannot guarantee to deliver positive results to each and every patient on whom they perform these procedures. There are numerous variables to be weighed: health, age and skin elasticity all play a large part in the outcome of the procedure.

Facercise is a natural alternative to cosmetic surgery. The process is risk-free and the results are predictably beneficial. It's like going to the gym regularly. If you do the exercises, you are going to see favourable results. Facercise also provides a safe and effective way for an individual to overcome almost any genetic or emotional destiny. Many of my clients come to me because their mouths are starting to resemble their mother's. Holding on to stored emotions, stress, anxiety and just the normal wear and tear of life can alter a person's physical appearance dramatically. The Facercise exercises help to create a younger, more relaxed-looking face. One of my clients stated, after being taught the mouth and lip exercises, 'I am no longer my mother. Now I am myself.'

As you do the exercises, you'll learn to use your facial muscles in a controlled manner. People tend to consistently overuse certain muscles, resulting in deep, unsightly expression lines. For example, when someone is in a confrontational situation, their demeanour is *always* tense. Think about it for a moment. If you are upset about something and you are questioning why someone did what he or she did, you will most likely conjure up your 'confrontation face'. You'll furrow your brows. You'll tighten your forehead muscles and get that face on. Over the years this can have an adverse effect on your face. After learning the Facercise techniques, however, you will gain control over these muscles and you'll use your face (and your muscles) in a more relaxed state. You won't create more expression lines or deepen the ones you've already developed. As one of my clients said to me after a private session, 'Facercise does it all.' By 'all' she meant toning and tightening the face, improving the texture and colour of the skin, smoothing out the fine lines, brightening the eyes, and relieving stress and tension, leaving her with an overall energetic appearance.

My clients

MY CLIENTELE RANGES in age from late teens to way past what a ninety-two-year-old client refers to as her 'middle earlies'. I get numerous letters and cards from young people, some in their teens, whom you wouldn't expect to be interested in facial exercises. However, even young people can have facial problems and surgery most probably is not the appropriate solution for them. Their problems range from faces that just lack tone to faces that are too wide or too narrow. Some have facial problems as a result of dental work, accidents, birth conditions and surgical operations. Here are some excerpts from young clients of mine:

☑ Lancy Coffer, a twenty-three-year-old from Holland, writes, 'I was in really poor health and for some reason I lost the muscle tone in my face. I started Facercise and couldn't believe the quick results. It worked and I was only out the price of your book.'

☑ Tom Zane, a twenty-one-year-old from Dallas, Texas, writes, 'I was hit by an eighteen-wheeler and had five bones in my face broken. Facercise relieved the numbness and coldness in my face.'

☑ Peggy Greene, a twenty-two-year-old from Beverly Hills, writes, 'I have a round face and a double chin. I feel I am too young for surgery. I started using your facial exercises after I read an article in Women's World, referencing Candice Bergen doing facial exercises and your programme. My face has become more narrow. My friends tell me I look like I've lost weight.'

My not-so-young clients have sent me similar letters.

☑ Ian Weeler, a seventy-two-year-old from Germany, wrote to me, 'I had major reconstructive jaw surgery on my upper and lower jaw to correct a severe misalignment. The surgery was muscle invasive. As swelling goes away, you are left with sagging facial muscles which have forgotten what to do. They took six inches of bone out of my face, which left me with excessive skin, which needed to be toned up. With your exercises, I'm gaining control of my muscles once again and everything is moving back where it belongs, instead of falling down to my neck.'

☑ Janice Mande, a fifty-eight-year-old from Great Britain, writes, 'I was involved in a traffic accident and suffered a whiplash injury. I had tried chiropractors, acupuncturists, everything. Within a week of doing the neck and jaw exercises, I noticed a dramatic improvement in my neck. This is miraculous, since every practitioner assured me they had done all they could and I would simply have to live with things as they were.'

☑ Sandy Rindlis, a sixty-two-year-old from Canada, writes, 'I had cataract surgery on my left eye and the surgery messed up my left eyelid. It didn't open as wide as my right eye. I also had Bell's palsy which left one side of my face tired looking. With your exercises, I have evened out my eyes and they can equally open and I've toned and strengthened my face so the remnants of Bell's palsy are no longer visible.'

Benefits of Facercise

These testimonials point out that exercising the facial muscles has important therapeutic and restorative as well as cosmetic benefits. I stress this to all of my clients continually. It's just so obvious. These exercises work and can sometimes perform miracles. I'm always amazed when I read an interview or an article by someone in the medical profession who states empirically that there is no scientific evidence that facial exercises work. Tell that with a straight face to my millions of clients who have seen, first-hand, the invalidity of that kind of comment. Tell that to Dr Wilma Bergfeld, MD, a past president of the American Academy of Dermatology, who stated 'those who call exercising facial muscles heresy aren't using the available medical knowledge about the effect on overlying structure when you make muscles larger.' On that subject, I can still vividly remember watching Jack LaLanne, America's foremost body fitness guru, talking about facial and body exercises on his TV shows in the 1950s. While other kids my age were watching *Howdy Doody* and *I Love Lucy*, I was watching Jack's exercise programmes. I was in agreement with his philosophy about exercises. It made absolute sense to me then, just as it does now. On his web site, Jack states, 'I was forty years ahead of my time. The doctors were against me, but I knew more about the workings of the muscles in my body than most doctors.' He's eighty-seven at the time of writing, and he looks fabulous. The medical profession hammered him all those years ago, ridiculing him and stating that there was no scientific evidence that exercising the muscles of the body really worked. Really! Those who criticize facial exercise, whether in the medical profession or the media, remind me of a comment made by Christopher Morley. He said, 'A critic is a gong at a railroad crossing, clanging loudly and vainly as the train rolls by.' Tell it like it is, Chris.

Many in the medical field are more enlightened, however. According to Dr Wilma Bergfeld, 'Exercising facial muscles in a reasonable fashion *certainly* [my italics] can improve the general appearance of the skin's surface without harming it in any way.' Dr Gerald Walman, an Arizona ocular plastic surgeon, said, 'Facercise is a carefully researched and scientifically developed method of exercising individual facial muscles and sets of muscles. I saw that these exercises can and do effect positive changes in tightening and firming the upper and lower eyelids.' And Beverly Hills plastic surgeon Dr Lawrence Birnbaum has stated that 'logic seems to dictate that good facial exercises would prevent many of the ageing manifestations'.

Success worldwide

I have been instructing on Facercise techniques for over two decades now. I've watched it develop from a skincare clinic in Monterey, California, to become a worldwide phenomenon. It's been an exciting time and continues to be more so every day. I am continuously expanding and improving the exercise techniques to afford the maximum benefits to anyone who is willing to work the programme. I travel throughout the world, giving seminars and promoting the numerous benefits of my techniques. I've taught socialites, rock stars, royalty, celebrities, politicians, athletes and business leaders throughout the world. I've given seminars for beauty professionals at the University of London and been a guest speaker at the Les Nouvelles Esthetiques congresses in France and England. I was the keynote speaker at the international Women's Club in Brunei, and I have lectured at the Health and Beauty Conference in Hong Kong and at the Nova Estetica in Argentina. I've been a guest speaker for selected audiences in Jordan and was also guest speaker at a charity benefit for *Harpers & Queen* magazine and Emporio Armani in London.

I have instructed professionals to teach Facercise in beauty spas in Europe, Asia, the Middle East and North, Central and South America and now have licensed instructors in six countries. My first book, *Carole Maggio Facercise*, has been a bestseller now for years in many countries and has been translated into eleven different languages. Facercise itself was voted one of the world's top one hundred beauty aids by *Harpers & Queen*. I've appeared on numerous television and radio shows throughout the world as well as being written up in magazines and periodicals such as *Harpers &*

Queen, Marie Claire, Vogue, Elle, Town and Country and the *New York Times*. When I began my career, the majority of my clients were women. Now, however, the men seem to be as concerned about their appearance as the women. That's great because men can benefit from these exercises just as much as women. Facercise is designed to enhance, tone and tighten individual facial features. There are fourteen essential exercises and nine progressive exercises. You don't need to do the whole programme in one sitting. It's a flexible, adaptable routine. The exercises can easily be merged into anyone's busy day, no matter how busy you are. For example, you can do the Eye Enhancer while sitting at a traffic light. You can perform the Nose Shortener while talking on the phone and the Cheek Developer while sitting at your computer. Facercise is the most user-friendly facial exercise programme ever invented. You don't need anything other than what God gave you to do these exercises. No gloves, no masks, no electronic stimulators, no electricity, no mirrors and, best of all, you can do them anywhere. You're the boss. Consider this book your personal trainer for your face and your mirror will provide you with glowing progress reports and all the encouragement you will ever need.

I take 'before' and 'after' photographs of my private session clients. I have thousands of these photographs collected over the years. The camera tells a story and the camera doesn't lie. There are visible changes evident after just a few days of doing Facercise. Do

The bad news as your face ages

✘ Skin becomes grey and sallow

✘ The nose continues to grow longer and wider

✘ The lips grow thinner

✘ Upper lip lines appear

✘ Eyebrows and eyelids droop

✘ Under-eye puffiness increases

✘ The jawline sags and jowls start to develop

✘ Nasal labial lines appear

✘ The mouth corners start to turn down

✘ The chin sags and a double chin starts to develop

✘ The skin on the neck grows loose and crepey

The good news as you Facercise

✔ Skin tone becomes more rosy and glowing

✔ The nose shortens and narrows

✔ The lips become more full and sexy

✔ The eye brows and eyelids raise

✔ The under-eye puffiness diminishes

✔ The jawline firms and the jowls tone up

✔ The nasal labial lines soften

✔ The mouth corners turn up

✔ The chin tones and the double chin recedes

✔ The skin on the neck tightens

✔ Increased blood circulation and oxygen flow throughout the skin and facial muscles will bring about a rapid change in the muscle tone, colour and texture of your skin.

You'll be amazed, pleased and very satisfied. If you devote eleven minutes, twice a day, to Facercise (in your home or your car) for at least five days a week, you'll see very definite results. You'll also probably have people asking you if you've recently cut your hair, lost weight, changed your make-up or are just back from a vacation.

Most of the world seems to be more exercise focused today. We are willing to work our bodies hard with exercises for an hour or so a day. We know that this is good for us. So why have we neglected the face? Helen of Troy is said to have had the face that launched a thousand ships. Why let Helen hold a record like that? Why not let Facercise launch a *million* new faces, yours being one of them?

Facercise will counteract the gravity's pull on your face. You are in control. Each day you will be able to see how you are making great strides in holding back the ageing process. You *can* turn back the clock and slow down the hands of time.

Facercise has given me profound professional and personal fulfilment. It is an absolute privilege to share my programme with you. I can tell you, without reservation, that if you do Facercise exercises properly, you will see and feel tremendous changes in your face as well as your self-esteem. Remember that the mind is the most powerful tool you possess as a human being. Use this tremendous tool to improve your face and your life.

yourself a favour. Take a picture of yourself before you start, both front and profile shots, and then do the same thing in ten days, using the same pose and, preferably, wearing the same make-up. Don't smile for either set of photos. You be the judge of those results.

2

How does Facercise work?

GOOD BONE STRUCTURE, great cheekbones and a sculpted toned jawline are facial features we all wish we had. Most people would credit good bone structure as the key component of facial beauty, but few people realize what an important role muscles play in moulding the contours of the face. Without facial muscles you couldn't blink, smile or frown. The face would just be a mask. Since the muscles in the face are smaller (and thinner) than most other muscles in the body, they react more quickly to an exercise regime. Because the fat-to-muscle ratio in the face is lower than it is in most other parts of the body, if they are exercised properly facial muscles can develop quickly. This can very rapidly give your face more definition and tone.

Some muscles in our body get exercised whether or not we mean to exercise them. We don't voluntarily have to exercise our legs, arms or hands, for example. They get exercised when we get out of bed and continue to get exercised until we get back into bed. We don't use our facial muscles like that. These muscles need to be exercised specifically if we want our faces to look as good as they should. Picture the stomach of someone who never works out. Not a pretty picture, is it? Now picture the stomach of someone who exercises that area consistently. Notice a difference in your mind? Of course you do. The same principle applies to our faces. We don't have to like it, but we all subconsciously know that, when muscles sag, the skin attached to the muscles also sags. Slack facial muscles are the primary cause of sagging and drooping, bags under the eyes, pouches and unsightly jowls many of us have as we get older. Lack of facial exercise also allows the muscle tissue to become thin and atrophied. This

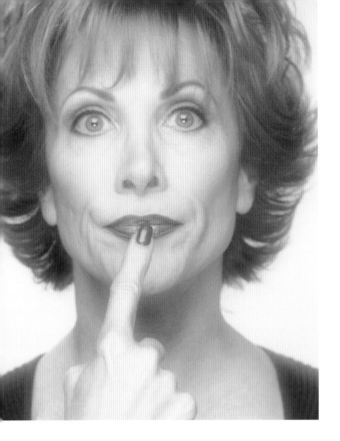

makes a person look old. It was George Burns who said that 'you don't have to be old to look old'. That's a very true statement.

Many of us neglect our facial muscles and probably hope for some magic cream or exotic elixir to magically appear on the market to help us correct our facial woes. Creams can improve the texture and appearance of the skin, much the same as make-up can improve the visual appearance of the skin, but there is no cream, no magic potion of any kind that can improve the muscle tone or lift the facial muscles, no matter what you read to the contrary. As Dr Albert Kligman, a well-known research dermatologist, has said, 'Facial sagging cannot be pharmacologically corrected.' Creams and topical lotions won't prevent the eventual sagging of your face.

There is an alternative to looking old, however, and

I'm sharing it with you in this book. Isolating and working the muscles in the face to the point of feeling a lactic acid burn is what makes the Facercise techniques so effective. This tingling, burning sensation occurs when a muscle is exercised to capacity. The muscle produces lactic acid as a result of the expenditure of energy. It has used up ATP (adenosine triphosphate), a nucleotide present in all living cells that is vital for energy production. Exercise physiologists and personal trainers are very familiar with this process. They call ATP 'the energy molecule'. That, in a nutshell, explains the 'lactic burn'. Feeling this burn tells you that the muscle is working to full capacity and will grow stronger and larger. This process restores the muscle tissue, elasticity and tone, resulting in plump, stronger facial muscles.

Muscles are fibrous masses of tissue, which are composed of protein. Exercising these muscles promotes the thickening and strengthening of muscle fibres. You need to work the muscles until they tire to assure maximum results. Remember Jane Fonda's mantra, 'No pain. No gain?' Well, that's correct. The more a muscle contracts (the pain), the more it grows (the gain). It's also important to remember that after the muscle tires, rest is essential so that the muscle tissue can regenerate and grow larger. It's also important to eat enough protein in the diet to ensure muscle growth. Fish and eggs are a tremendous source of protein, as are red meat, turkey and chicken, and they are easily accessible. (See Nutrition, p. 107). With the right balance of exercise, rest and protein, the muscles adapt to the demands placed on them, producing beneficial results. By isolating facial muscles and performing repeated exercises, the muscles are strengthened, regenerated and enlarged.

Unique programme

Facercise is different from other facial exercise programmes. And here's why. Facercise will educate you on how facial muscles work. I'll also explain how the programme works. You'll learn to isolate the specific muscle groups in your face. You'll also learn physical and mental tools for resistance so that you'll be able to work your facial muscles to maximum capacity while you are doing other things at the same time, like working on your computer, driving your car or even watching TV. Best of all you won't need all the props most other facial exercises programmes require – no mirror, mask, white gloves or tricky finger placements. And you won't have to allot twenty-two minutes of 'quiet time' to perform Facercise exercises.

Some of the other facial exercise programmes have you doing a whole host of bizarre antics. Sticking out your tongue and gasping five times, or moving a ball of air from cheek to cheek, behind the upper and then the lower lip. Now I don't know about you, but if I'm going to perform this procedure, I want to know why it works. Alas, many of these exercise programmes

provide no logical explanation as to how they work. You just need to have blind faith, I guess. Imagine how many people have used uninformed exercise methods over the years? I remember those so-called fat-reducing, vibrating machines from the 1970s. Do you know *anyone* who *ever* lost weight from using one of those? How about those large, roller-like drums that you had to sit on? The rollers were supposed to reduce fat and inches. They didn't. They just thrashed you incessantly. The end result? They just made your bottom sore, bruised and probably bigger (from swelling). Doing something just because someone else says it works isn't enough for me. I want to know *how* and *why* it works. If standing on my head will add years to my life, I'll do it, but only if it's explained *how* and *why* it will extend my time on this planet.

To obtain the results you'll want and you deserve, you need to remember that there are no 'quick fix' methods. In these health-conscious times, most of us are aware of what we need to do if we want to build authentic muscle and reduce body fat. A low-fat diet, a cardio-exercise programme and a carefully devised weight-training programme are the ticket. No short cuts will work effectively over the long haul. You also have to do all of these things continually. To build body muscle you need to do multiple sets of repetitions with weights to pump the muscles to create size and strength. Facercise is the first facial exercise programme to apply these same techniques to the face. With Facercise, you pump the cheek muscles, for example, in the same way you work out to give yourself muscular, defined legs.

Since I started teaching facial exercises, I have always continued to consult plastic surgeons, dermatologists and physiotherapists in order to constantly refine the exercises and make them as effective as possible. Facercise won't overdevelop your facial muscles. It *will* tone and define them.

The effectiveness of Facercise

I've been asked on numerous occasions whether Facercise workouts will deepen wrinkles or stretch your skin. Actually, just the opposite occurs. As you exercise, you increase blood circulation to the muscles and other areas of the face. This results in firmer muscles and taut skin. The skin smooths out and the wrinkles are less visible. While Facercise cannot permanently restore or regenerate lost collagen, neither can cosmetic surgery. Collagen injections are painful and costly, can leave scars and must be administered every few months to maintain the puffed-up look they're designed to achieve. Facercise will greatly improve your skin tone from the inside out, unlike cosmetic surgery. And without the ouch factor.

One of the key reasons why Facercise is so effective is that it makes use of two of our most readily renewable assets – imagination and energy. Your mind and your energy play crucial roles in making Facercise work effectively. I call it the 'mind-muscle connection'. When I coach my clients, I tell them that they must feel their muscles working and they need to visualize their muscles growing with every repetition. Also, as you do the Facercise exercises, you are asked to focus on the lactic acid burning sensation in the facial muscles. This is an indication that you are performing the exercises properly, and with such a powerful physical feeling on which to focus, your mind will stay on track and you'll feel the muscles grow as you work towards achieving your goals. Your thoughts are just as powerful as your actions because you are seeing, as well as feeling, your muscles grow and strengthen as you progress.

This book will teach you fourteen essential and nine progressive facial exercises that isolate and work the fifty-seven muscles in the face and neck area. A network of fibres connect the face and neck muscles, so every muscle benefits from the exercises.

As you do the exercises, you'll be rewarded with a revitalized complexion. However, my Facercise exercise programme provides much more than the short-term benefits you'll see immediately. Exercising your face for twenty-two minutes at least five days a week will give you a lifelong youthful appearance. I'm fifty-six at the time of writing, and I can honestly say that my face is smoother, firmer, rosier and younger looking than when I was thirty-six, when my ex commented on my 'looking older than my age'. Since then, I've lost a lot of wrinkles along with the person who suggested that I had them and I have the photographs to back up that statement.

Before and after

The picture on the left was taken when I was thirty-six. That's pre-Facercise. My face was wrinkled from years in the Arizona sun, as I mentioned earlier. I had a thin, gaunt look because of collagen loss, just one more collateral result of the sun damage I had experienced during my youth. My eyebrows were sagging and tired looking and my eyes looked smaller than they were because my upper brows and eyelids were drooping so much. No amount of make-up could hide my under-eye bags. My complexion was grey and sallow and not as youthful and glowing as I would have liked. My cheeks were low and flat on my face and I had an overall tired look. In a nutshell, I looked older than my years. Sound familiar?

Now have a look at my most recent photo (right), taken at the age of fifty-six. My wrinkle lines are much less visible. I have high, full cheeks. My face is wider and smoother and my eyebrows have lifted. My eyes are open and large. My skin tone is much more youthful and peachy. I can't tell you how many times people have asked me, 'Who did your cheek implants?' When I tell them I did, they look very sceptical, until I demonstrate by pumping my cheek muscles for them. I also have a better-looking nose now, because I've built up the muscles in my nose. (Yes, your nose does have

muscles.) As for my lips, they no longer appear low and thin but have a fuller and more youthful shape. The corners of my mouth have turned up, giving me a younger, pert look.

I always present my before and after photographs when I appear on TV shows to talk about Facercise. I like to tell the story about a woman in the audience at one of these shows. She stood up and announced, 'I don't see any difference in those before and after photographs.' I told her, 'Thank you. I considered that a tremendous compliment because the pictures were taken over twenty years apart.' She signed up for a Facercise class on the spot.

Clients have told me that one of the most exciting moments to occur after they start Facercising is when they actually start to *feel* the muscles under their faces. The sensation encourages them because they can tell the exercises are working. They are conscious of that usually dead area between the cheekbones and the mouth or the space between the ear and nose. It's kind of like how your legs feel the day after you've started an exercise programme. You'll notice something different. You'll feel a little sore. It's minor muscle ache, but that's a good sign. If the feeling is uncomfortable, you can alleviate it by blowing between your lips, which disperses stored lactic acid in the muscles just as stretching leg or arm muscles helps you feel better after you've exercised those areas.

I am extremely proud to be able to offer people

such a healthy, easy, effective programme to improve their facial appearance. Facercise is effective for numerous reasons and one of them is that these exercises are actually fun to do. By making faces for a few minutes each day, you can restore youth and vitality to your countenance. Facercise is an easy, enjoyable method for renewing your beauty. The exercises are also effective stress busters, which relax your face, body and mind. Are there any other benefits as well? Yes, indeed. You don't need any props. Need more reasons to Facercise? How about this? One of my clients told me that she had a much younger man come up to her as she was doing a face-narrowing exercise in her car. He thought she was flirting with him. She found him attractive. That's one way to start up a conversation.

Before and after

Below: pre-Facercise, aged thirty-six.

Right: aged fifty-six, with dramatic facial changes.

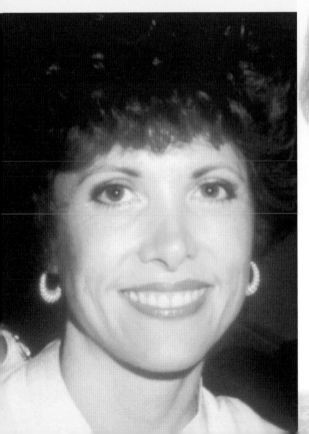

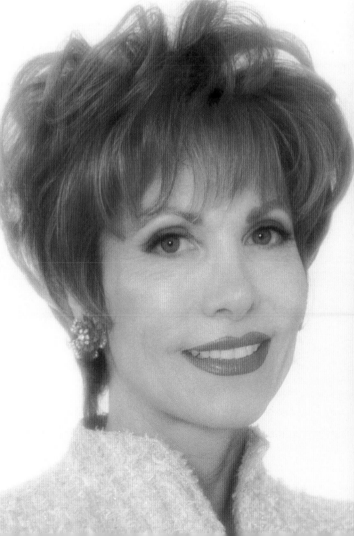

3

Let's 'face' it

How to pinpoint and understand your unique facial features

Most people's self image is inexorably tied to their physical appearance. According to *Self* magazine, eighty-five per cent of women in the United States don't like their bodies. Imagine how many of those women also don't like their faces. What's the status of *your* self-image? How do you *really* feel about your face? Be honest here. There are probably features that you do like. But how about the features you don't like or would like to change? Virtually no one has a completely flawless complexion and beautifully proportioned features. Heredity plays a major role in determining our facial features and bone structure. Cosmetic surgery can alter your facial features but Facercise is going to improve your facial features naturally. The change Facercise is going to make in your face will be as exciting as it is fantastic. When Winston Churchill said 'there is nothing wrong with change, if it is change in the right direction', he was right on the money. A positive change in your face is definitely a change in the right direction.

It's vitally important that you become familiar with your face before you initiate any exercises. You may feel that you're an authority on your face, sometimes too much of an authority. I want you to be acutely aware of your face's pleasing features as well as your facial flaws. It's also going to be important to understand the reason for your facial flaws. This knowledge will be indispensable as you work toward correcting those flaws. It'll also help you note the progress you make as you move along.

Becoming a student of your face's weak points and the way it has aged may make you a bit uncomfortable, but you must have a *realistic* picture of your face before you start your exercise programme. Remember people in the limelight – celebrities, models, entertainers, politicians, royalty, business leaders, movie stars, you name it – all had to confront their flaws. They had to be realistic. So do everyday people. I did. Remember my botched nose job? So, let's make a start: assess the beauty of your face honestly and impartially. Doing this will give you a realistic approach as you travel toward positive improvements.

A photograph or two will help you honestly assess your face. How many times have you looked at photos of yourself at work or at play and said to yourself or out loud, 'I don't really look like that, do I?' The answer to that is, 'Yes, you do.' The good news is that you can do something about what you see in those photos. Mae West once said that 'Too much of a good thing is a good thing.' I like to think she was referring to Facercise. Keep in mind that it is important to know how you really look, not how you think you look. Remember that our mind can play tricks and we can't always count on it to be honest. But you can really count on the camera to be honest. When I give my seminars, I always take a Polaroid picture of each person in attendance so they can study their facial features during my lecture. I've found that most of them become *very* attentive after a few minutes of study. I remember one woman who returned to the sign-up desk, picture in hand, and said, 'You've given me the wrong photo.' I looked at the photograph she held and said, 'This lady has the same blouse and earrings as you.' She said, 'I didn't realize that I had two chins.' The

picture she held was the judge and the jury and I rested my case then and there. A photo will be blunt and honest. It will show you how your face really looks to others; not how you think it looks. Remember how the mind can play tricks? That's important to keep in mind.

Have two photos taken, one profile and one front view. And remember – *do not smile*. You want to see how the muscles look when they're relaxed. Your face will definitely look different from how it appears in the mirror. Remember, the camera doesn't lie. Make written notes when perusing your features from the picture. Are my eyebrows too low? Do I like the shape of my nose? Is my face narrow or wide? Are my lips full or too thin? After you've exercised your face for several weeks, take two more photos, front and profile. Have the same expression and take the pictures from the same distance. You want to compare apples with apples here. Study the photos carefully. See how many changes you've been able to make in this short time period. Eyebrows lifted? Lips fuller? Face wider or narrower? Are the wrinkles less obvious? Any changes in the nose? Make some new notes and continue the exercises. Keep defining and refining your face. Your face will continue to make positive changes as long as you continue to exercise. When you make up your mind to really stick with the Facercise programme, your face will reap huge dividends. Just fully commit to the exercises. As I like to say, 'Do it big, or stay in bed.'

Lines and wrinkles

Every face has lines. Even a day-old baby has lines and wrinkles. Without them, a face has no expressive quality and looks blank and lifeless – like a mask. Also like some people who have had too much cosmetic surgery, perhaps. In your late twenties, your face is maturing along with your mind and body. All three of these things work in harmony to form the appearance one presents to the world. By the time we enter our thirties and beyond, our faces have acquired some lines and wrinkles. Mark Twain once said, 'Today's wrinkles are yesterday's smiles.' He was serious about that, I'm sure. That's why he changed his name and wore a bushy moustache. I would like to rephrase that by saying 'yesterday's smiles *don't* have to be today's wrinkles'. Not if you Facercise. And let's not forget that there are different types of facial lines. Not all wrinkles are lines and vice versa. It's a fact. By understanding how these lines differ from each other, you will be able to objectively study and know your face.

■ **Built-in lines** These are lines formed by expressions and habits. Many are hereditary and they help to give the face an individual character. Some people question things in their lives so frequently that they have what I call the 'question mark' lines between their brows. Other people squint habitually, which gives them crow's feet faster than you can say it.

■ **Sleep lines** These are the lines I like to refer to as the 'night-time enemy'. Face muscles are working even while you sleep; insidiously and relentlessly creating skin lines and wrinkles without you even knowing it. And if you're one of those people who bury your face in your pillow when you sleep, you'll eventually make Rip Van Winkle look like he was just born yesterday.

■ **Lines due to collapsed muscles** The stomach isn't the only part of the body to sag visibly as the body grows older. The facial muscles begin to collapse as well if they are not properly exercised. This will cause many new lines to form in the skin.

■ **Scar lines** These lines are the result of injury, infection or disorders of the skin. By toning the facial muscles, facial exercises can help to restore the natural elasticity of the skin, improve circulation and create a smoother appearance.

■ **Sun damage fine lines** If you've spent years in the sun (as I did), you're going to have fine lines from all that sun bathing when you were younger.

Factors affecting the skin

If you consume a lot of alcohol and caffeinated drinks, such as coffee, tea and cola, and rarely drink water to flush out your system, you could have a whole host of skin problems. Mild dehydration contributes to bags under the eyes, sallow skin, blemishes, acne and numerous other ailments of the complexion. I know W.C. Fields was once quoted as saying that he never drank water because of the disgusting things fish did in it, but let's never forget that drinking water is an excellent way to keep the skin clear, rosy and smooth. Let's also never forget that our bodies are seventy per cent water and never forget, too, that W. C. Fields drank plenty of other things to get his complexion to look the way it did.

While your energy level, personality and emotional make-up influence your facial appearance, you can't forget that heredity still plays a major role in facial features and bone structure. As you study your face, you will, no doubt, notice some things you've inherited from your ancestors and the older we get the more pronounced these features become. We start to resemble our mothers and fathers. Check out their features. Do you want to look like that? You may or may not. If you don't want to resemble those individuals, you can re-route or at least delay Father Time's inexorable journey across your face. Physical traits can definitely be passed down from generation to generation. Did your father furrow his brow when he was under pressure? Did your mother purse her lips when things weren't going smoothly? Did someone in your family grimace or frown or distort their face when the stress thermometer was turned up high? If any of these sound familiar, relax. Don't stress. Doing Facercise can help counteract these inherited traits. Just keep working on it and be conscious of the traits in the first place. And speaking of mothers, let's not forget what the playwright Florida Pier Scott-Maxwell once said: 'No matter how old a mother is, she still watches her middle-aged children for signs of improvement.' Don't worry, Mum. You're going to see some real improvement in your kids. And soon, because they are reading this book, which means they're going to be Facercising shortly.

Continue to study your photographs as you progress. Make up your mind about what you feel are your plus and minus attributes. Which features do you wish to accentuate? Which features do you want to play down? Be objective. Look at that face in the photograph and focus on the changes you want to make. Write them down. Do your Facercise exercises regularly and see how dramatically you can change those facial areas you wish to change.

Seven days of Facercising

Take a look at the truly dramatic results achieved by the people in these photos after just seven days of Facercising. Imagine what the results would be after one month.

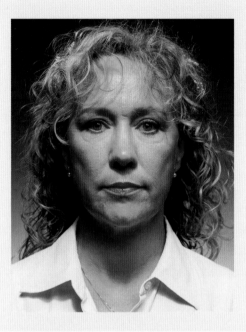

First day

Barbara exhibits an overall lack of muscle tone and a dull complexion. She has drooping eyelids, under-eye puffiness, heavy nasal labial folds, tight thin lips and a weak jawline.

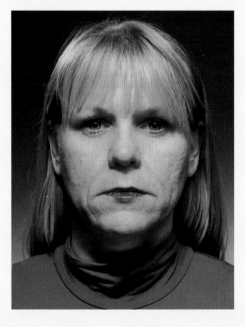

First day

Brenda has an acne-scarred, chalky complexion and heavy eyelid hooding. Her cheeks are low and flat, her mouth corners have turned down and her lips are thin and wizened.

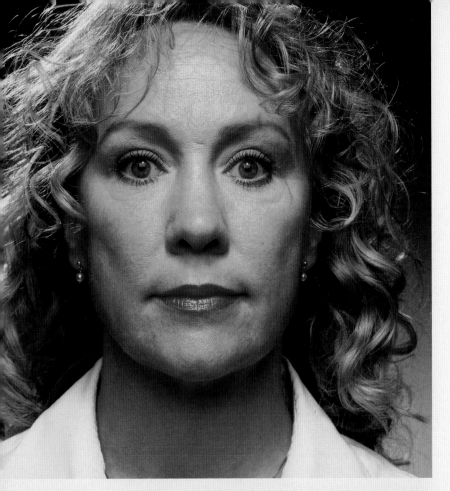

Seventh day

Barbara's overall muscle tone has greatly improved. Her complexion is glowing, her eyes have opened dramatically and her under-eye puffiness has greatly diminished. Her nasal labial area has softened, her lips are more full and sexy and her jawline is more defined.

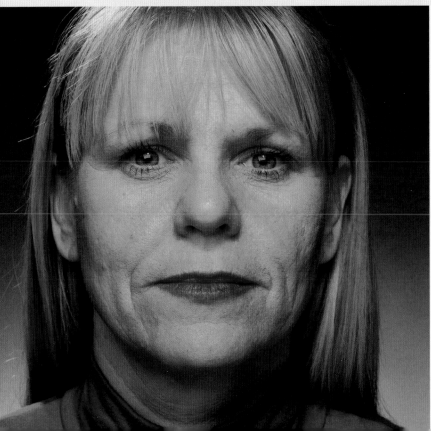

Seventh day

Brenda's complexion now shows a more rosy tone and her acne scars are less visible. Her eyes have opened up and her cheeks are higher and fuller. Her mouth corners have turned up and her lips are much more full.

First day

Linda has heavy eye hooding, a dull complexion and an overall lack of muscle tone, with a heavy jawline.

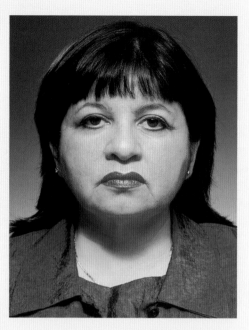

First day

Princess exhibits heavy hooding on her eyelids, hollows under the eyes, heavy nasal labial fold, a slack jawline and a double chin.

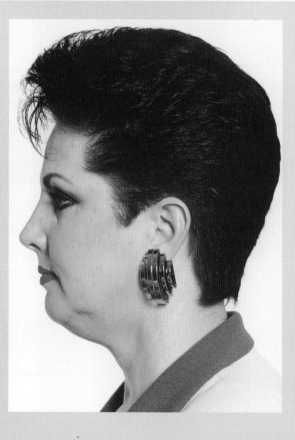

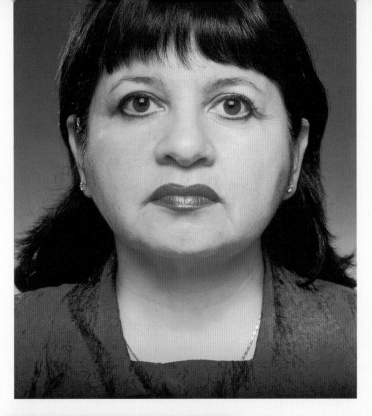

Seventh day

Linda's eyes have opened considerably. Her complexion is much more alive and vibrant. Her face has an overall uplifted look.

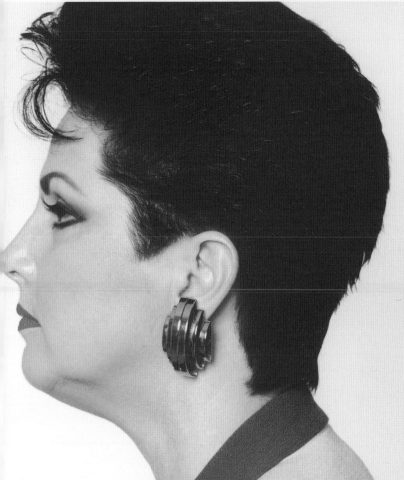

Seventh day

Princess's eyebrows and eyelids have lifted and her cheeks have also lifted, filling in the hollow under her eyes. Her nasal labial area has smoothed out and her jawline is more defined. Also, her double chin is less apparent.

The seven signs of ageing

Here is a summary of the seven main signs of facial ageing:

1. Low eyebrows

When the muscle tone around the eye weakens, the area under the eyebrows begins to look low and heavy. This is especially true with the profile. By doing the Forehead Lift (see p. 56), you will strengthen the muscles around the eye and scalp muscles so that the brow is lifted naturally. You'll also strengthen the tiny vital muscles in the eyelids, keeping the entire eye area smooth and youthful.

2. Drooping eyelids

Take it from me, even if you're a drop-dead gorgeous movie star or a fresh scrubbed beauty, there is no escaping drooping eyelids as you age. I'd love to tell you this isn't true, but it's a fact of life. Remember what I said in Chapter 1? Eyelid surgery is the third most popular plastic surgery procedure performed today. Drooping or heavy eyelids can be a family trait or just the cruel rewards of age. If you look at the picture of me at thirty-six on p. 27, the hooding of the eyes made me look older than my years. The Eye Enhancer exercise (see p. 52) will strengthen the upper eyelids so that the muscles become stronger and the eyes open to appear larger and more rounded, giving you that youthful look we all would like to have. Your eyes will be more vibrant and seem more alive.

3. Low, flat cheeks

Here I'd like to introduce you to the Big Three facial enemies: **Heredity**, **Age** and **Gravity**. It's no fluke that the acronym for these three scourges is HAG. These nuisances work tirelessly together to create cheeks that appear low and flat on the face. As cheek muscles atrophy, the face begins to lose its curves and it begins to flatten out like a tabletop. It's not a pretty picture. This joint effort by HAG creates a tired, aged appearance. The Cheek Developer (see p. 58) can build and plump up the muscles so that the cheeks appear higher on your face. They look sculptured and full. When my clients feel their cheek muscles move, they are excited because they know they are making headway. After several weeks the enlarged, strengthened cheek muscles will give your face a firmer, more defined appearance. You're going to like what you see. Relegate HAG to the back burner indefinitely with Facercise.

4. Nose faults

Remember Pinocchio? He was a little boy puppet who magically came to life, but when he told a lie, his nose would start to grow. When we get older, we don't have to lie to get our noses to do this. It just happens naturally. As cheek muscles slacken and sag, a hollow area starts to develop around the sides of your nose. While gravity pulls the nose down, the muscles around the mouth gradually begin to lose their shape and their tone. This double whammy contributes to sagging. To keep your nose looking young and firm, you need to develop the tiny nasal muscle located under each nostril. By doing the Nose Shortener (see p. 62) daily, you'll improve the appearance of the nose as well as the upper lip. I *know* this works. I was able to do this to sort out my botched nose job.

5. Thin, lined, hard-looking lips

As we age, the lips and the surrounding areas start to become thin and wizened. Tension, smoking, the sun and habitual facial expressions are the causes of this condition. This is no beauty gain, ladies and gentlemen. And since no one likes dried-up withered lips, we need to do something about this because the resulting lined, sunken effect can add years to a person's appearance. By performing the Lip Shaper (see p. 66) and Lip Line Smoother (see p. 102), you can rebuild the muscles around the mouth and say goodbye to the wizened look. Welcome aboard, fuller, more sexy lips and softer upper lip lines.

6. Sagging jaw and/or double chin

Heredity plays an important part in the shape and tone of the jawline and chin, as I've mentioned before. George Orwell once remarked that by the age of fifty, everyone had the face they deserved. He was off by about twenty years. Actually, by the age of thirty or so, your jawline and chin can start to sag, droop and lose definition and tone, which results in a weak, aged appearance. You can greatly improve the firmness and tone of your jawline by doing the Jaw Strengthener and the Neck and Chin Toner. A strong and defined jawline gives a person a sense of confidence and assurance. Don't be one of those people to whom Groucho Marx was referring when he said, 'I never forget a face, but in your case I'll be glad to make an exception.'

7. Crepey lined neck

We've all seen people, even relatively young ones, with creased or crepey-looking throats. That may be suitable for a turkey but it's not a look we find particularly attractive. This look is usually caused by too much sun and/or lack of exercise, coupled with plain old ageing. Since the skin on the throat is thin, it exhibits age more quickly than on other areas of the body. If the neck is thin and the muscles are not in tone, then this look is exacerbated. By exercising the neck area using the Neck Strengthener and Neck Toner exercises (see pages 70 and 78), you will learn how to restore the shape and size of the neck muscles and smooth the skin. This will greatly improve the appearance of the entire throat area.

Facial faults checklist

Now that you've studied your 'before' photographs and have had a chance to reflect on the pluses and minuses of your facial features, it's time to get busy. Remember that you can't help getting older but you don't have to *look* old. The writer Anthony Powell once said that growing old was like being increasingly penalized for a crime you didn't commit. That's a cute sentiment but I have a remedy for that. You have the power to do something about the ageing process and I'm going to unleash that power in you through Facercise. On the following checklist, mark off the features you want to improve. Don't be shy or coy. Go for it. Once you have completed the checklist, you will have a record of what you are going to correct with Facercise. You'll have the 'before' and 'after' photographs to chronicle the amazing journey you are about to take as you gradually rebuild your face to accommodate the new you. Seeing is believing and the pictures are going to make believers out of all of you.

Jackie completed her checklist and Facercised for seven days. Her positive changes are impressive and will become more so in the following weeks.

First day

Jackie has heavy eye hooding and heavy under-eye puffiness. Her cheeks are low and flat on her face. She has a very apparent nasal labial fold and her lips are actually receding into her face.

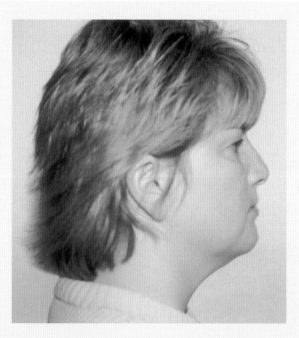

Low eyebrows ☐

Droopy eyelids ☐

Long, flabby, or enlarged nose ☐

Low, flat cheeks ☐

Thin, lined, hard-looking lips ☐

Turned-down mouth corners ☐

Saggy jawline ☐

Double chin ☐

Crepey, lined neck ☐

Now that you've had a chance to examine your face and ticked your areas of concern on the checklist, you've earned a rest. Take a few minutes to think about all the positive changes you are going to make in your face. Don't worry if you've ticked all of the problem areas. You're just being honest and guess what? You're not alone. Hope Blance once said, 'I hope I look as good as my mother does when I reach the age she says she isn't.' I always get a chuckle out of that. I chuckle because I know that Hope's mother probably does Facercise and has for all those years she says she doesn't have. So take a break now. Just don't go out and sit in the sun or put your face in a pillow.

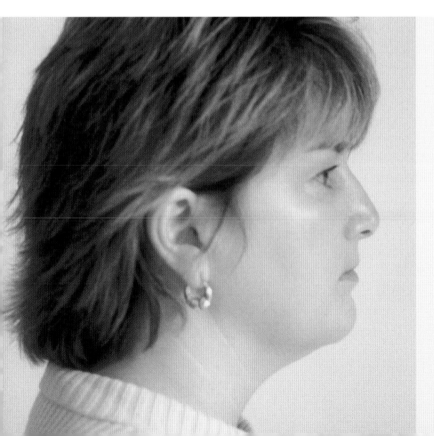

Seventh day

Jackie's eyes have opened and the under-eye puffiness is greatly reduced. Her cheeks are higher and appear more full. Her nasal labial fold has virtually disappeared and her lips are more full and pouty.

4

Muscles of the face and neck

Where they are, what they're called, how they work

MOST PEOPLE HAVE a general understanding of the muscles of the body and how they work. They also understand that certain exercise programmes will keep these muscles strong and toned. Millions of health- and age-conscious people have already started a body exercise programme. They are pec-pumping, stair-stepping, treadmilling, jogging, ab-crunching, aerobic dancing, you name it. They know that these exercises will quickly develop a better-looking body. Few people, however, have any understanding of their facial muscles, what they are called and how they work. So, for all of you who took anatomy classes in school because you needed the sleep, here's a refresher on what you missed.

The human face has fifty-seven muscles which work together to support and maintain the facial features. With every facial movement you make, from furrowing your brow to laughing at a joke, or even quickly downing that doughnut before anyone sees you, your facial muscles are synergistically working to perform myriad functions.

Possessing a working knowledge of the facial muscles and being able to picture their location and capabilities will assist you in creating the mind–muscle connection which is so important to successful facial development. This is the core of Facercise: you will be consciously using your mind to exercise your facial muscles. Your exercise programme will be successful because it is built on decades of rock-hard Facercise experience.

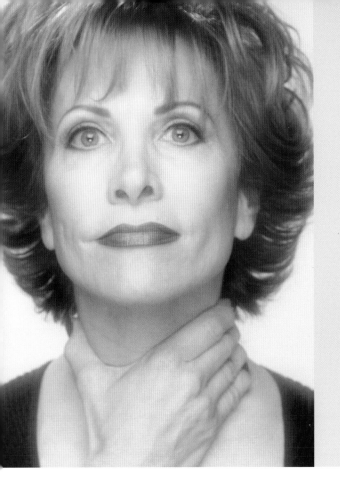

When you begin to learn the Facercise exercises, you'll feel your facial muscles move and flex, just as you would if you were exercising your biceps or calf muscles. Facial muscles resemble a patchwork quilt lying just beneath the surface of the skin. These thin layers of muscles are interconnected with bundles of fibres. I consider these muscles magical because of the artistic feats they perform. Working with connective fibres, these muscles give your face life, animation and all the expressions that make us unique. Without these acrobatic muscles, our faces would be mask-like.

Facercise hones in on all the muscles in the face, neck and scalp. The muscles are interconnected, so they are all working together. When you begin your Facercise regime, it's essential that you do the exercises in the order in which they are given in this book. When you initiate an exercise, you are working a particular group of muscles in the face. When you move on to the next exercise, the first group of muscles begins recuperating and rebuilding. Being aware of the facial muscles and using your visualization powers to expand the muscle's activities (seeing it get larger or feeling it move) are all part of the Facercise concept of mind–muscle connection. You'll need to focus and concentrate to remain in this state of mind. If you do this, you'll start to see some amazing changes in your face in a short period of time. The longer you do the exercises, the better the muscle memory will be and the more effective the exercise becomes. Take a few minutes to study the muscle groups as described on the next few pages. Possessing a rudimentary working knowledge of your facial muscles, their location and what they do will definitely help you in bringing your best face forwards.

Muscles of the scalp

The skin of the scalp is the thickest skin on the human body (which might account for the term hard headed).

■ Beneath the skin are a number of scalp muscles, including the *epicranius*, which raises the eyebrows. It is divided into different areas.

■ The *frontalis*, which is part of the *epicranius*, is a thin muscle located over the forehead. It raises the eyebrows and the skin over the root of the nose and simultaneously draws the scalp forwards, throwing the forehead into transverse wrinkles. In layman's language, it is responsible for frowning. The Forehead Lift strengthens the frontalis, lifting and toning it, keeping forehead wrinkles from forming.

■ The *occipitalis* measures about three and a half centimetres (an inch and a half) long and lies at the back of the head. It is also part of the *epicranius* and draws the scalp backwards. The entire scalp may be moved forwards and backwards by the activity of this group of muscles. Again, the Forehead Lift enhances the *occipitalis*, providing the same results it achieves with the *frontalis*.

■ The *galea aponeurotica* is a broad, flat tendon that covers the upper part of the cranium, joining the *frontalis* and *occipitalis* muscles. It too benefits from the Forehead Lift.

Are we having fun yet?

Muscles of the mouth

■ The *orbicularis oris* completely encircles the mouth. It consists of numerous strata of muscular fibres, which travel in different directions and connect with fibres in the upper and lower lips, cheeks, nose and the surrounding areas. This muscle affects the closure of the lips. The Lip Shaper and Cheek Developer are great exercises for firming and toning it and, consequently, for improving the appearance of the lips.

■ The *buccinator* is a broad, thin muscle at each side of the face beneath the cheek. It assists in the act of sucking. The Cheek Developer and Face Slimmer work wonders for the *buccinator*, helping to tone and strengthen it.

■ The *mentalis* is a tiny muscle in the front of the chin. It raises the chin and makes the lower lip protrude (pout) and it also wrinkles the skin of the chin. The Lip Shaper exercise will firm up this muscle, resulting in a firmer, fuller lower lip, without those costly and temporary collagen injections.

■ Next in line is the *triangularis menti*. This triangular muscle rises from the lower jaw up to the mouth and it helps to draw down the corners of the mouth (watch it in action when you pout, or when you're upset, or when your mouth starts to resemble your

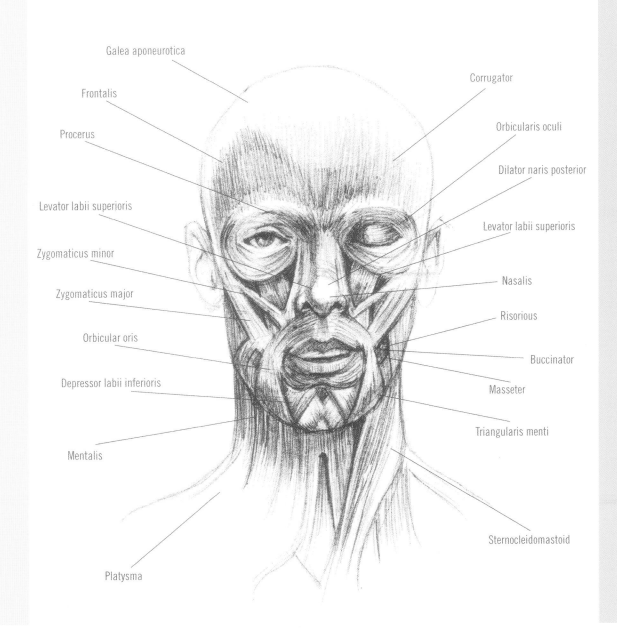

Galea aponeurotica

Corrugator

Frontalis

Orbicularis oculi

Procerus

Dilator naris posterior

Levator labii superioris

Levator labii superioris

Zygomaticus minor

Nasalis

Zygomaticus major

Risorious

Orbicular oris

Buccinator

Depressor labii inferioris

Masseter

Triangularis menti

Mentalis

Sternocleidomastoid

Platysma

mother's). By doing the Mouth Corner Lift, you'll tone the corners of the mouth, which will keep the mouth corners from turning down.

■ Another muscle to benefit from the Mouth Corner Lift is the *risorius,* a narrow bundle of fibres, widest at its origin. This muscle varies quite a bit in size and form. It is involved in smiling, acting to retract the corners of the mouth towards the back teeth.

■ When you laugh, you use the *zygomaticus major* and *minor.* These are two slender muscles comprised of cords of muscle fibres that draw the angle of the mouth backwards and upwards. Again, the Mouth Corner Lift will work wonders here.

■ Next up is the *quadratus labii superioris.* This is a broad sheet of muscle that lies around the upper lip and is connected to the cheek muscle. Its function is to raise the lip (snarl). The Lip Shaper and Face Energizer are just the ticket for this muscle.

■ The *quadratus labii inferioris* is a small quadrilateral muscle that draws down the lower lip (into a mini pout). The Lip Shaper will help to keep this muscle firm and toned.

■ The *caninus* raises the upper lip to form a sneer. Keeping this little guy in shape is a job for the Lip Shaper.

Muscles of the nose

■ First we have the *procerus.* This pyramidal muscle crosses the bridge of the nose. Its function is to pull down the middle of the eyebrows and it produces transverse wrinkles over the bridge of the nose. Not an attractive picture, is it? The good news is that the Nose Shortener exercise will help counteract the effects this muscle produces.

■ The *nasalis* begins at the bridge of the nose and extends upwards over the bridge of the nose, compressing the nostrils. The Nose Shortener strengthens this muscle.

■ The *depressor septi* extends across the base of the nose and closes the nasal openings by pulling down the septum (the cartilage partition between the nostrils). Practising the Nose Shortener will help tone the muscle and keep the nose from growing longer and/or wider.

■ The *dilatator naris posterior* is next on the list. It lies near the margin of the nostril and it acts to increase the size of the nasal opening allowing more air into the lungs. Working this muscle can help to recontour the shape of the nose.

■ The *dilatator naris anterior* is a thin and delicate muscle, which lies directly above the middle of each nostril. This muscle opens the nostrils, causing them to flare.

It's important to understand that all the muscles of the nose work closely together. The Nose Shortener benefits them all in different ways.

Muscles of mastication

These are the muscles used in the opening and closing of the jaws, for example in chewing or yawning. Many people hold the tensions of the day in their jaws. Knowing the location of these muscles and how to work them can help you to alleviate these tensions and relax, as well as building up the muscle tone in your face.

■ *Masseter* and *temporalis* are muscles that work in conjunction with each other to close the teeth with force, as happens when you chew food or gum. They also collaborate to grind your teeth in your sleep.

■ Next up we have the *pterygoideus externus*. This short, thick muscle is somewhat cone-shaped. It assists in opening the mouth and rotating the jaw.

■ The *pterygoideus internus* is another thick, quadrilateral muscle. It contributes to the crushing, grinding action of the jaw.

The Jaw Strengthener is the *exercise du jour* here. It exercises all of the above muscles and helps to keep them toned, defined and firm. No slack jaw here.

Muscles of the eye

■ The *orbicularis oculi* is a powerful muscle that surrounds the orbit of the eye. It acts involuntarily, closing the eyelids gently, as when you sleep or blink. When the entire muscle is brought into action, the skin moves in folds, which radiate out from the outer corners of the eyelids. These folds form those infamous 'crow's feet'. The Eye Enhancer exercises this muscle without creating folds in the skin.

■ The *levator palpebrae superioris* is a thin muscle in the upper eyelid. It maintains the firmness of the upper eyelid, keeping it from drooping. The Eye Enhancer will help keep this muscle toned and taut and will help you maintain that youthful, open-eyed look.

■ The *epicranius* is the muscle that raises the eyebrows. Exercising this muscle increases oxygen and blood circulation throughout the forehead and eye areas. Regular exercise of the *epicranius* can soften your brows and give you a more relaxed appearance.

'The eyes are the windows to the world.' That's how Dr Gerald Walman, Medical Director at ImageCare Laser Center in Scottsdale, Arizona, so poignantly puts it. He correctly points out that the eyes are probably the most important part of the face because when people meet they are drawn to each other's eyes. Eye contact is the first thing any successful person needs to develop if they are going to succeed in the business world. Any rejuvenation of the eyelid area has got to be the number one most effective way to improve our image.

Dr Walman once told me that he was impressed at the variations in the muscle tone that could be observed with the passage of time and how this muscle tone directly related to the aesthetics of the facial area. He went on to state that individuals over forty usually exhibit an increased loosening and laxity of the eyelid tissues, generally caused by loss of elasticity in the underlying tissues which are supported by the *orbicularis* muscle. This loss of elasticity leads to bulging of the fat pads within the orbit surrounding the eyes, resulting in bags under the eyes. This loss of muscle tone also contributes to wrinkles and crow's feet. Dr Walman should know. He has over twenty-two years of experience in ophthalmology and ocular-plastic surgery. He also stated to me that regular facial exercises that work the *orbicularis* muscle and other facial muscles surrounding the eye area *will* increase tone and thus decrease the severity of wrinkles, crow's feet and other problems that afflict the delicate skin surrounding the eye. What can I say? The doctor knows best.

Muscles of the neck

■ The *platysma* is a broad, thin plane of muscular fibres lying under the skin on each side of the neck. It is a powerful muscle and it produces oblique wrinkles in the neck and depresses the lower jaw. The Neck Toner and Neck Strengthener are excellent exercises for toning and honing this muscle so that the skin smoothes out over the neck area.

■ As well as being a very long word, the *sternocleidomastoid* is the muscle that rotates the head and turns it to either side. This is a fairly large muscle, which is thick, broad and very powerful. The Neck Toner and Neck Strengthener exercises work very well on this muscle to keep it toned and strong.

■ The *trapezius* is located at the back of the neck and shoulders. It turns the head from side to side and works in tandem with the *sternocleidomastoid*. The Neck Toner and Neck Strengthener exercises work on this muscle as well, with equally positive results.

Muscles of the ear

There are three small muscles, which lie right under the skin surrounding the ear. These muscles have very little effect on facial appearance but they are interconnected to other muscles that Facercise uses to have a *big* effect on the overall toning and honing of the face. It is very important to learn how to make these little muscles move so as to achieve optimum results in strengthening and defining your scalp and facial muscles. When you are doing exercises designed to firm up your jawline, for instance, concentrate on flexing your ears. This will help you focus on the jaw muscle groups and will enhance the exercise. Additionally, when you are doing exercises which lift and tone the upper eye and eyebrow area, flexing the ears will help ease frown lines around the eyes.

■ The *anterior auricularis* is the smallest ear muscle. Thin and fan shaped, it assists in drawing the ears forward. When you are doing the scooping movement in the Jaw Strengthener exercise, remember to concentrate on flexing the ears.

■ The *superior auricularis* is the largest of the ear muscles. Its function is to raise the ears. While this movement may seem almost non-existent, when you are doing the Face Narrowing exercise, concentrate on this muscle. You should visualize your ears lifting as you visualize the sides of your face moving up. Don't be discouraged if you don't see or feel it move. It is the visualization of the muscle movement that assists you in exercising the surrounding muscles.

■ The *posterior auricularis* draws the ears backwards. When you are doing the Face Widening exercise, imagine pushing your ears backwards as you mentally expand the sides of your face. This will help you to visualize the sides of the face widening. It's this action which actually makes your face wider and fills in the gaunt, drawn area of the lower face.

Ready to begin

Now that we've introduced the main players in the face, it's time to put them to work for you, not against you. You're ready to introduce your face to Facercise, which is about to change the way you look at yourself and the way others look at you.

Photographer Barbara Colson once said, 'It's not wrinkles. I just have too much skin for the size of my face.' Sorry, Barb, but wrinkles are wrinkles. The good news is that we don't have to get rid of that extra skin. We just have to tone it up. Facercise does exactly that.

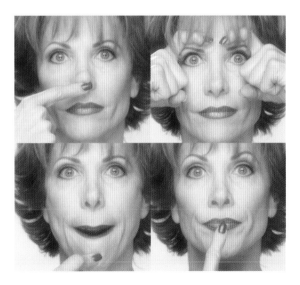

Facercise is going to be your ticket for a fantastic journey – a journey which is going to result in a more attractive, younger looking you. So, all aboard. This is one trip you are not going to want to miss.

5
Let's Facercise

Fourteen essential exercises

Facercise is a two-part programme. In this chapter you will learn the fourteen basic exercises. You'll gradually perfect these through daily practice. Consistency is the important concept here. As you keep practising, these exercises will become second nature in a matter of weeks and you will start to see the changes you were hoping to achieve. As your face starts to change, becoming more sculptured and defined, you will want to move on to Chapter 6, where you will be introduced to Progressive Facercise. These are exercises that will further enhance the toning and tightening which is so important to overall facial development. Be sure to learn the fourteen essential exercises first, so that your muscles are in shape for the progressive techniques. When Benjamin Franklin advised that 'you have to walk before you can run,' he was on the right page. As you master these exercises, you will find yourself automatically doing them because they make your face feel so alive and vibrant. You know how you feel when you've just done something very good for yourself? Well, that's the feeling I'm describing.

As with any important part of your daily regime, you need to schedule Facercise into your routine from the very start. A good way to begin your day is to do each of the fourteen Facercise exercises once, which should take up about eleven minutes of your morning. You can even do this while lying in bed. It's a great way to wake up. These exercises will enliven you and help reduce night-time puffiness. Your face will look more toned and defined as you put on your make-up, giving you a more attractive appearance. What's wrong with that? In the evening, I suggest you do each set of exercises again, for eleven minutes. This way you'll get in your two sessions daily and your face will be relaxed and ready for a good night's rest. If you're like most

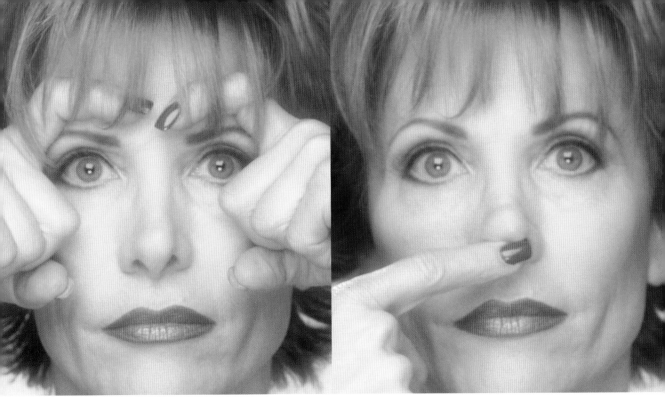

people I know, you're living your life in the fast lane. Time is important and no one I know has enough of it. It's important that you allow yourself the time to do constructive things for yourself, however, so I have developed a sequence of exercises that can be done even while you are driving your car to work or shopping.

To obtain the results you will want to achieve, you'll need to do the exercises twice daily for six to eight weeks, while you are in the learning stage. Most of my clients find that after a few months of disciplined workouts, they've knocked from five to ten years off their appearance. Once you have achieved the initial benefits you started out to obtain, you'll probably want to move on to a maintenance programme or take the next step up and start practising the Progressive Facercise exercises (see Chapter 6). Do the exercises as your face needs them. Don't rush. Trust your mirror.

Remember that since you've started the Facercise programme the mirror is now your friend.

Have fun with Facercise. It's going to be your most valuable facial treatment. Read through all the exercise directions two or three times before beginning the programme. While you are reading about the exercises, visualize yourself actually doing them. You are right around the corner from achieving that younger, vibrant face your mirror has been telling you that you don't have yet. Remember that mirror? You may not have been too happy with it lately but you *will* learn to love it very soon. Trust me.

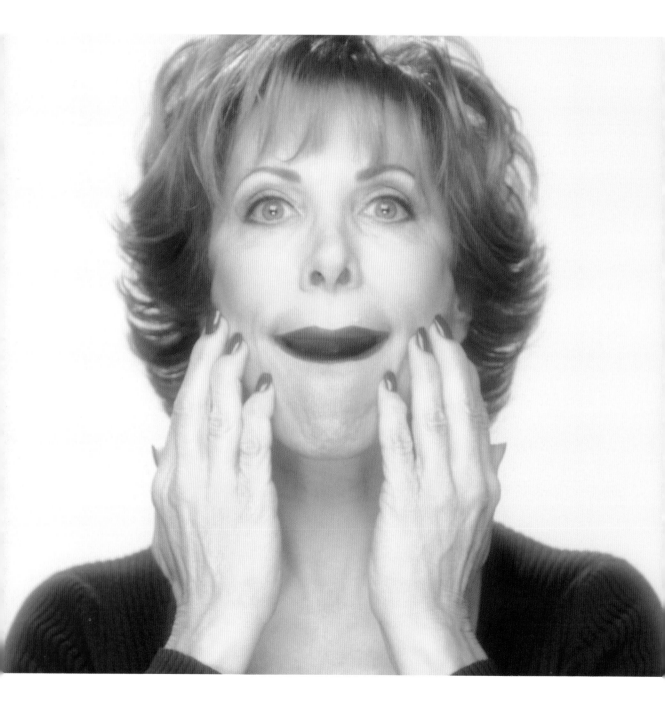

Four tips for success

1. Posture As you prepare to do each exercise, pull your navel back towards your spine, as far back as you can. Wrap (tighten) the front of your thighs around toward the back of your thighs and tighten your buttocks. Hold this position while you do the exercise. This posture acts as an anchor and will allow you to focus on the individual facial muscles you are exercising. A very pleasant side effect of this exercise, many of my clients tell me, is that their hips actually get smaller. Anyone interested in that? *Now, remember:* each time you see the words 'assume the basic posture' as you read through these exercises, I want you to assume the position defined above. This is the position that will best enhance these exercises.

2. Lactic acid burn Concentrate on the muscle group you are working until you feel that tight, achy feeling. The exertion creates a build-up of lactic acid in the muscle and the burning sensation is a sign that the muscle is being worked to its maximum capacity. Remember, no pain, no gain. The fingertips are your counterweights in facial exercising. They provide the resistance necessary for the muscle to work harder, grow stronger and achieve results as quickly as possible. I have a term I call 'pulsing'. Pulsing is moving your fingers quickly up and down on the muscle to intensify the lactic acid burn. Don't forget this term. You'll need to remember it always. It works.

3. Visualization Visualize and feel the energy coursing through your muscles as they work. Picture in your mind these muscles lifting and starting to move up your face. When you read through the exercises that follow, you will see that I often say things like, 'follow the energy in your face'. My concept of energy flow is based on the traditional Chinese medicinal theory that energy moves in pathways around the body. I know from experience that feeling and visualizing energy flows helps people learn the exercise techniques more quickly. The big pay-off is that visualizing energy leads to more rapid muscle development than exercises done without using your imagination.

4. Ache away To relax the muscles after the exercises, press your lips together and blow between them, making sure that you vibrate the lips. It's the sound you'd make if you placed your face in the bathtub and blew bubbles through your lips, like we all did when we were kids. You'll be doing this routine after each exercise to relax your facial muscles and 'blow away' the ache.

Exercise 1

The Eye Enhancer

Benefits

The Eye Enhancer exercises the *orbicularis oculi* muscle which surrounds the entire eye. One of the most important muscles in the body, this muscle opens and closes the eye. This exercise pumps blood into the total eye area and strengthens the upper and lower eyelids. This exercise also reduces under-eye puffiness, lifts under-eye hollows and, in effect,

Method

1. You can perform this exercise lying down or in a sitting position. Assume the basic posture (see p. 51). Place your middle fingers between your brows, above the bridge of your nose. Place your index fingers with light pressure at your outer eye corners. Look towards the top of your head. Make a strong squint *up* with the lower eyelid. Feel the outer eye muscle pulse. Squint up and release ten times while focusing on the muscle pulsing each time.

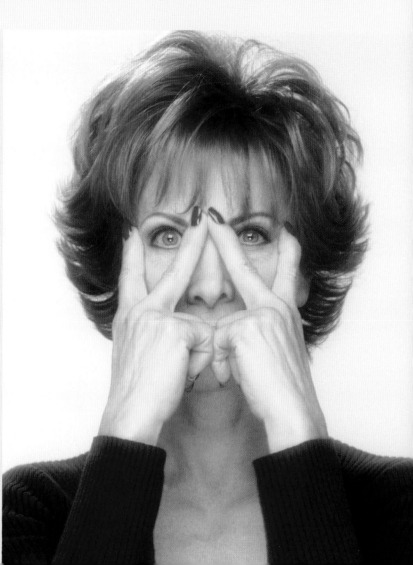

enlarges the eye socket, giving you a more wide-awake, bright-eyed look. How is that possible? Here are the facts. As you age, the upper eyelid muscles lose their tone and sag down on the eye socket, invading the area and making it appear smaller. By toning and lifting the upper and lower eyelids, the eye socket becomes more defined and appears larger.

Tip: Perform the Eye Enhancer twice a day. If you have deep hollows or severe under-eye puffiness, repeat the exercise three times daily. **Use slight pressure with your middle fingers, between the brows. This will not allow your eyebrows to furrow or wrinkle. Keep your index fingers at your outer eye corners, using light pressure so as not to create creases in your skin.**

2. Hold the squint and squeeze your eyes tightly shut, keeping your buttocks tight, and count to forty. It's *very important* to keep your eyes closed tightly and your buttocks tightened as you count.

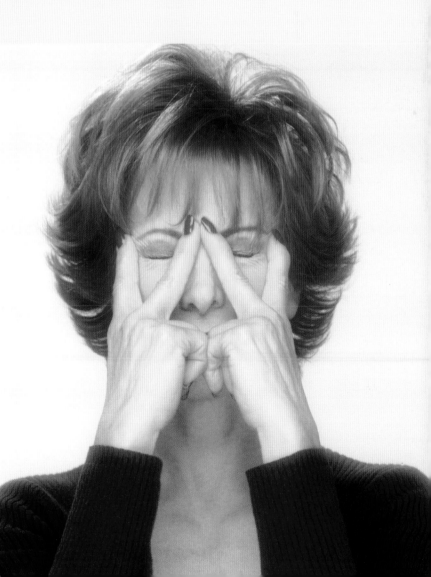

Exercise 2

The Lower Eyelid Strengthener

Benefits

This exercise also strengthens the *orbicularis oculi* muscle, firming the lower eyelid, diminishing the hollows under the eyes and reducing under-eye puffiness.

Method

1. You can do this exercise sitting up or lying down. I alternate positions to work the muscle differently. Assume the basic posture (see p. 51). Place your index fingers at your outer eye corners and your middle fingers at your inner eye corners and apply light pressure. Look up toward the top of your head. Make a strong squint *up* with your lower eyelids. You should feel your inner and outer eye muscles pulse. Squint up and release ten times, keeping your upper eyelids open wide.

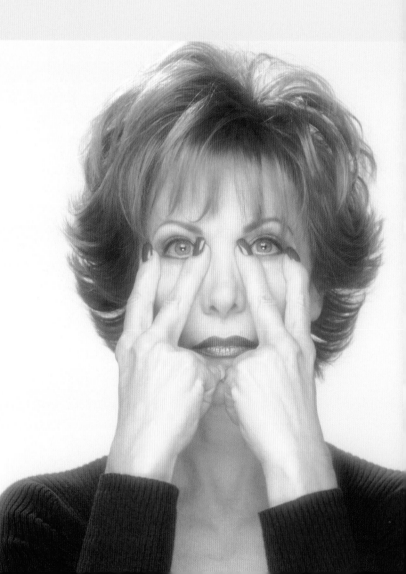

Tip: Perform the Lower Eyelid Strengthener twice a day. If you have extensive eye puffiness, repeat this exercise three times a day. Remember to keep a slight pressure with your fingers at the outer and inner eye corners to keep skin from creasing.

2. Hold this squint and think *up*, maintaining a strong squint with your lower eyelids. Remember to keep your buttocks tight. Count to forty, while focusing on the inner and outer eye muscles flexing.

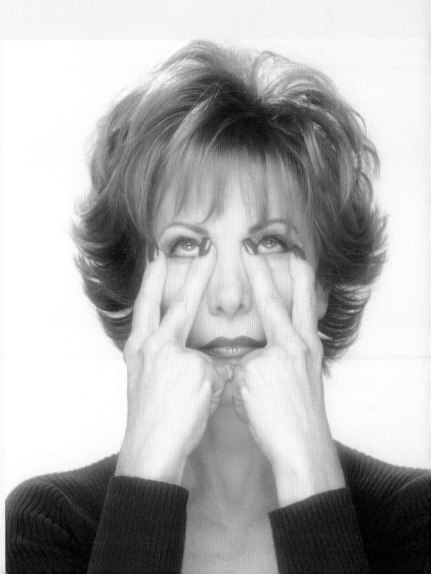

Exercise 3

The Forehead Lift

Benefits

This multi-purpose exercise works the *epicranius*, which raises the eyebrows, the *frontalis*, which draws the scalp forwards, the *occipitalis*, which draws the scalp back, and the *galea aponeurotica*, which joins the *frontalis* and the *occipitalis*. This exercise prevents or

Method

1. You can do this exercise in a sitting position or lying down. I personally like to do this one lying down because I feel that I can exert more energy. Assume the basic posture (see p. 51). Place the index fingers of both hands in the middle of the forehead so that they are parallel to the top of each brow. Now, pull the fingers down towards the brows. Keep them held down. Look up towards the top of your head. While you are pressing down with your fingers, concentrate on pushing the eyebrows up. Push them up and release them ten times.

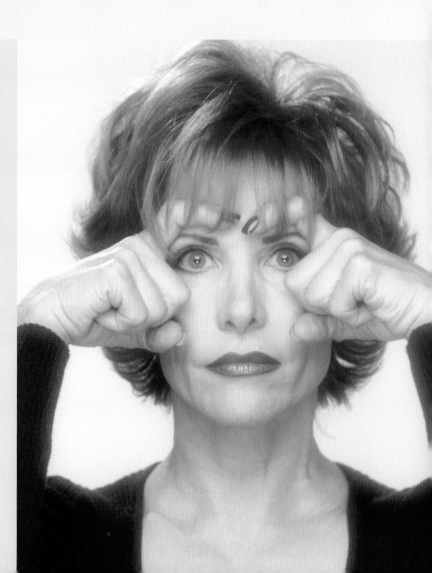

reduces the frown lines between the eyebrows and forehead and raises the eyebrows. It also acts to prevent or diminish the hooding effect that age and lack of muscle tone tends to cause on the upper eyelids.

Tip: Do the Forehead Lift twice a day. It helps to clear the head and will make you feel much more alert. To correct a heavy or scowling brow, repeat this exercise three times a day. If your fingers have a tendency to slip, use a piece of tissue, rolled up, under your index fingers for better traction.

2. Keep your eyebrows in the up position and continue to keep the fingers pressed down. Do mini-eye-brow push-ups until you start to feel a tight band of pressure above the brows. When you feel the pressure or burn, keep your eyebrows pushed up with your fingers pushing down against them and hold your brows up. Count to thirty. Release and massage the centre of your brow in circular motions. This will relax the muscle and result in optimum development.

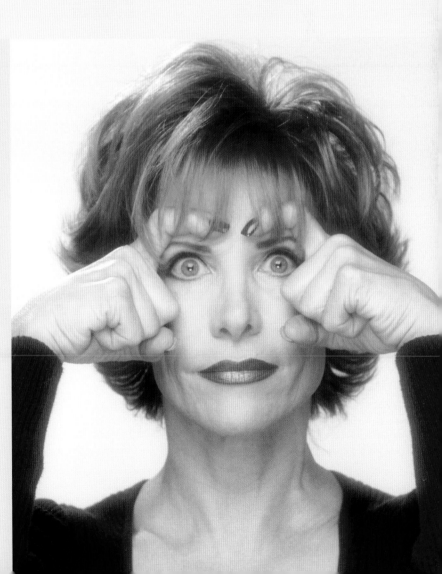

Exercise 4

The Cheek Developer

Benefits

The cheek developer exercises the *buccinator* muscle. This muscle forms the rounded top part (the apple) of the cheek. The exercise also works the *orbicularis oris*, which is the circular muscle surrounding the mouth. It lifts and enlarges the cheeks and removes hollows from under the eyes.

Method

1. This exercise can be performed while sitting, moving or lying down. I like to do this one sitting up because I feel I can get more of a 'push' out of it. Assume the basic posture (see p. 51). Imagine a dot in the centre of your upper lip. Imagine another dot in the centre of your lower lip. Open your mouth and pull the two dots apart. This should allow you to form a long, strong oval shape. Hold this oval shape firmly in place, keeping the upper lip pressing down against the teeth. Place your index fingers lightly on top of each cheek (the apple).

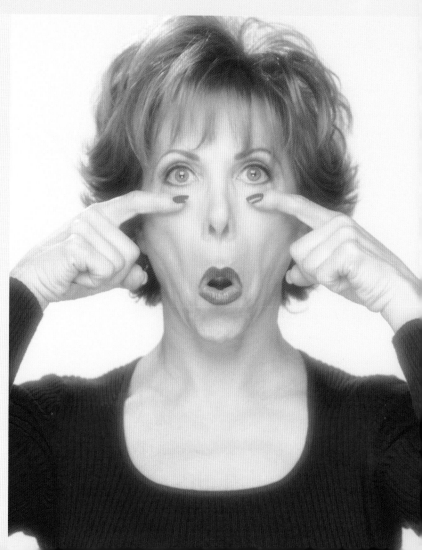

Tip: Perform the Cheek Developer at least twice daily. You can easily do this exercise while working on your computer, watching television or even walking around. If you experience an ache in the jaw area, you are using your jaw to smile and release the cheeks, not your upper lip. Use only the upper lip pressing down against the teeth. To alleviate an ache, blow between your lips. This little activity releases the lactic acid in the muscle and should immediately banish the ache.

2. Smile with your mouth corners and then release the corners. Push the energy up under the cheek muscles and repeat this movement thirty-five times in quick succession. Use your mind–muscle connection to visualize pushing the muscle up under the cheek each time you smile. You should feel your cheeks moving as you do this exercise. To enhance the movement, you can tighten and release your buttocks each time you smile and release with your mouth corners. Tightening your buttocks during this exercise helps you to push your cheeks harder.

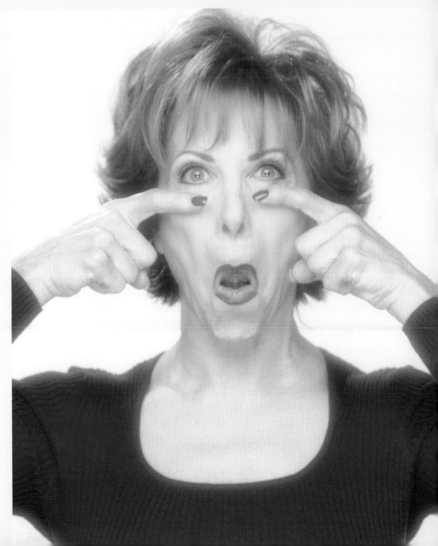

Exercise 5

The Face Energizer

Benefits

This exercise may look very similar to the Cheek Developer but there is one critical difference. The Cheek Developer makes cheeks appear higher and fuller while the Face Energizer works the *quadratus labii superioris* and uses the mind–muscle connection

Method

1. This can be done sitting up or lying down. I prefer lying down because I feel I can really push the stress out of my face from a lying down position. Assume the basic posture (see p. 51). Imagine a dot in the middle of your upper lip. Imagine a dot in the middle of your lower lip. Open your mouth, pulling those two imaginary dots apart, allowing your mouth to form an oval shape. Place your index fingers lightly on the top (apple) part of your cheeks. Smile with your mouth corners and release the corners. You should feel the cheeks move under your index fingers. Visualize pushing the muscle up under the cheek each time you smile. Repeat this movement ten times. On the tenth smile, use all of your strength to pull the upper and lower lip away from each other. Imagine that your cheeks are moving out from your face towards the ceiling, and then exiting, like two small balloons, out through the top of your scalp.

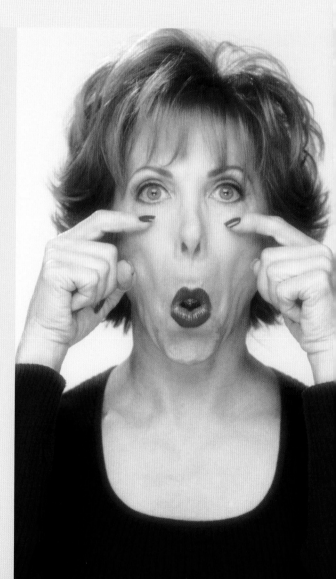

to counteract the lengthening and flattening effects of gravity. The Face Energizer removes the stressed look the face develops during the course of a busy day and increases blood circulation, giving your complexion a rosy, vibrant glow.

Tip: Do the Face Energizer twice a day. If you find that you are under unusual tension or stress, do it as often as you feel it is necessary. If you feel an ache in the jaw area after performing this exercise, blow out between your lips. This simple little act will release the lactic acid in the muscle and should give you an immediate feeling of relief.

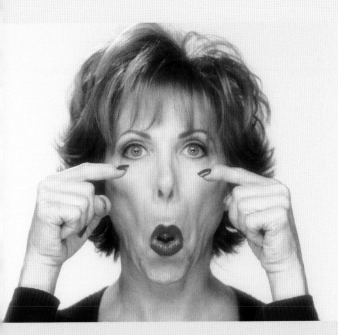

3. Now raise your hands above your head and raise your head an inch or so, lifting your head with the front of your neck and your tightened buttocks. Hold your head up, count to thirty and continue to imagine that the cheeks are moving out and up, exiting through the top of your head. Keep your hands outstretched above your head.

2. Take your index fingers and pull them half an inch away from your face and then move the fingers up in front of the face, towards the scalp area. This will help you visualize your cheeks moving up through the top of your head. Hold this position for a count of thirty, while looking up toward the top of your head.

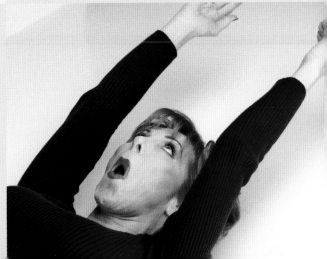

Exercise 6

The Nose Shortener

Benefits

The Nose Shortener properly stimulates blood and oxygen flow throughout the upper lip and nose area. Many of my clients have described a tingling feeling around the nose. This is good. It's a result of increased blood circulation to that area. That's what you want. As I've mentioned previously, our noses continue to grow throughout our lives. The tip of the nose drops

Method

1. You can do this exercise while on the move, or while sitting up or lying down. My preference is to do it while I'm on the phone. Push your nose tip up firmly with your index finger. Flex your nose down by pulling your upper lip down over your teeth or by pushing down on your nostrils. Hold for a second.

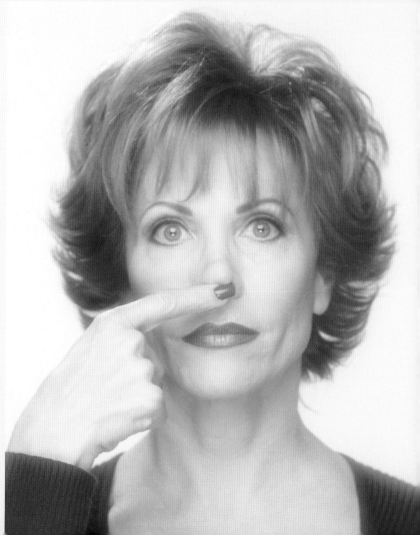

and widens with age. The good nose news is that this exercise shortens and narrows the nose tip by exercising the *depressor septi* muscle. Pinocchio should have read my book. He could have kept on fibbing and no one would have known. Politicians worldwide have been doing this exercise religiously for years because they all know it works.

Tip: Do the Nose Shortener once a day. If your nose is a little longer than you would like, or if it's a little too wide, perform this exercise twice a day. Some of my clients who have had rhinoplasty surgery reported that doing this exercise for several weeks helped to give their nose a more naturally sculpted look. I know this is true because it worked for me.

2. Release the lip. Repeat the exercise thirty-five times. You should feel the nose tip push against the finger each time. Remember to keep breathing at a normal rate while you perform these repetitions.

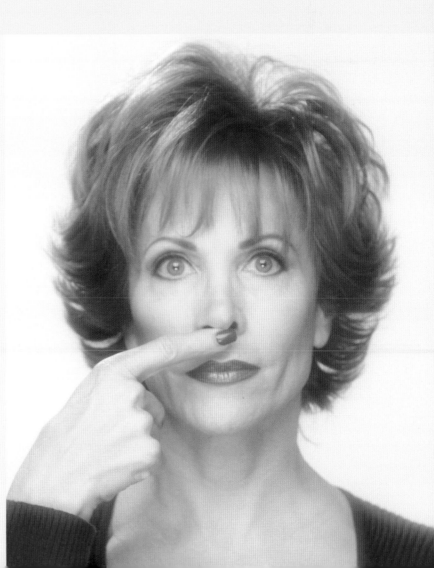

Exercise 7

The Mouth Corner Lift

Benefits

Unfortunately, as we age, the *zygomaticus* muscles sag, causing the mouth corners to droop. This exercise will firm those mouth corners and turn them back up in the right direction. This exercise can be done in pretty much in any position. I do it in the supermarket queue to kill some time.

Method

1. Press your lips together but do not purse them. It's more of an 'I'm resigned to it' kind of a look. Tighten the corners of your mouth into hard knots, as though you were sucking two small lemons toward the back teeth. Do not clench your teeth. Remember to maintain steady, normal breathing as you proceed. Place your index fingers lightly at the corners of your mouth. Keep sucking the corners of your mouth in as you visualize the corners of your mouth turning up into a tiny smile. Now visualize the corners turning down, resembling a tiny frown. Visualize turning the corners slowly up and down.

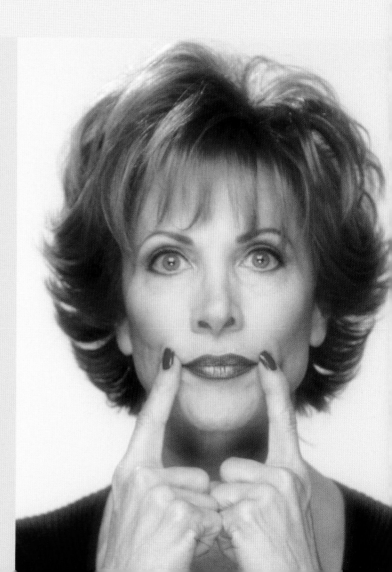

Tip: The success of this exercise hinges on your use of the mind—muscle connection. In your mind, you should be visualizing the corners of your mouth moving up and down, about half an inch, as you pulse the index fingers. This is a mental movement, *not* a physical one. You should do this exercise twice a day to keep your mouth from resembling your mother's.

2. Move your fingers away from the corners of the mouth in tiny up and down pulses. Visualize the energy in the corners. Continue to move the fingers away from the corners of your mouth in small up and down motions until you experience a burning sensation in these corners. Hold the burn feeling for a count of thirty, pulsing the fingers up and down quickly. This will intensify the burn. As you complete the exercise, you should feel that lactic acid burn. To release the lactic acid, blow through your lips.

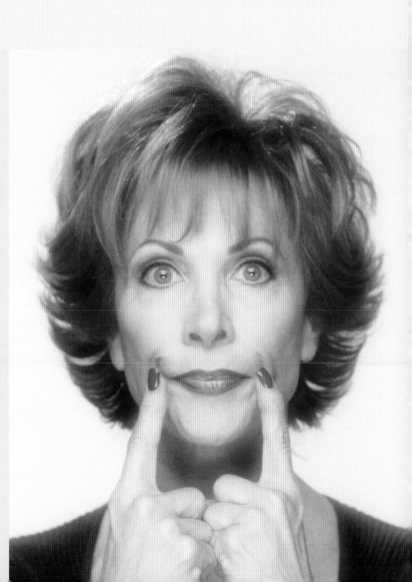

Exercise 8

The Lip Shaper

Benefits

By working the *orbicularis oris* muscle around the mouth, the Lip Shaper makes the mouth look younger, firmer and fuller. This exercise enlarges the lips and smooths out lines above the upper lip. I like to call this the 'no-collagen collagen' look.

Method

1. This exercise can be done either lying down or sitting up. I like to do it lying down because I like to lie down once in a while. Press your lips together, imitating your best pout. Do not purse your lips. Don't clench your teeth. Tap the centre of your lips with your index finger. Visualize crushing a pencil between your lips.

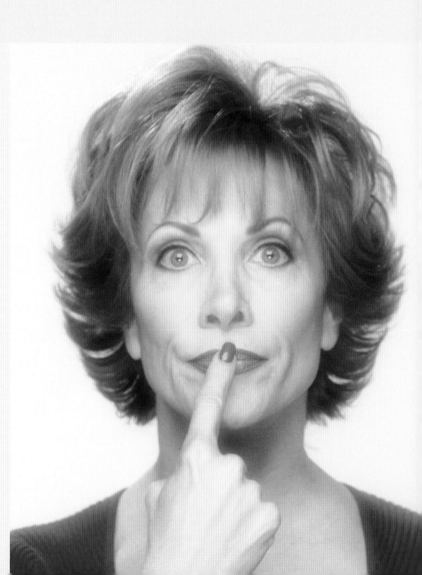

Tip: Do the Lip Shaper twice a day to plump up thin lips. This is a fabulous exercise for people who hold stress and tension in their mouth areas. Do not purse the lips, simply press them together. You should not see any creasing of the lip line.

2. *Slowly* pull your finger away from the centre of your lips. Visualize the pencil growing longer. Draw the energy point out and lengthen your imaginary pencil until you feel that burn. When you feel the burn pulse your finger up and down rapidly for a count of thirty. Release the lactic acid by blowing out through pressed lips.

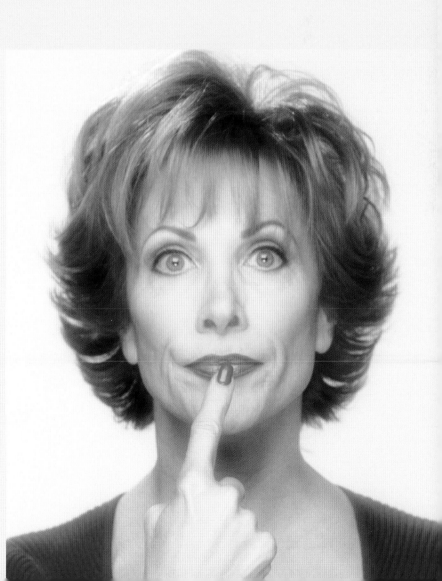

Exercise 9

The Nasal Labial Smoother

Benefits

This exercise can make a big improvement in your appearance. By building up the *dilator naris anterior* and the *dilator naris posterior* muscles, you will be able to plump out any deep creases and smooth out age lines from the nose to the mouth corners.

Method

1. This exercise is most effective when sitting in an upright position. Assume the basic posture (see p. 51). Imagine a dot in the centre of your upper lip and a corresponding dot in the centre of your lower lip. Open your mouth and pull the dots away from each other as you form a long, strong oval shape with your mouth. Remember to keep your upper lip pressing down on your teeth.

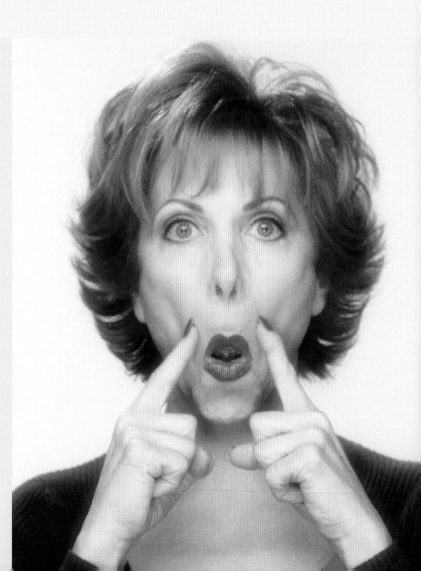

Tip: Using your mind–muscle connection helps intensify the burn and, consequently, develop the muscle more quickly. Do this exercise twice a day for optimum results.

2. Visualize a line of energy moving from your mouth corners up to the sides of your nostrils. Use your index fingers to follow this imaginary line upwards. Then visualize that energy beam moving back down the imaginary line towards your mouth corners. Now keep repeating this energy movement up and down and use your index fingers to intensify this imaginary energy. Keep this up until you feel the burn in the nasal labial line. When this occurs, pulse your index fingers up and down quickly to a count of thirty. Blow out between your lips.

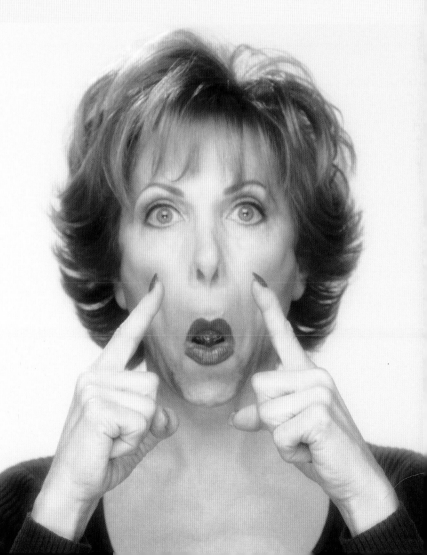

Exercise 10

The Neck Strengthener

Benefits

This exercise strengthens the *platysma*, the *sternocleidomastoid* and the *trapezius* which are muscles in the neck. These are very important strong muscles that allow us to hold our heads upright. Strengthening them will firm up and smooth out the

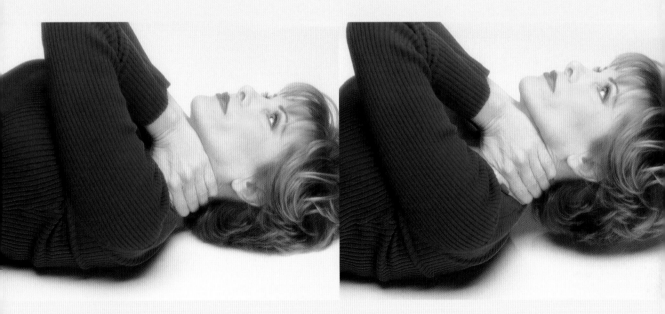

Method

1. The best position for this exercise is lying down. Assume the basic posture (see p. 51). Grasp the front of your neck with the palms of your hands as if you were choking yourself.

2. Lift your head about a centimetre (half an inch) off the floor, lifting with the *front* of the neck and your tightened buttocks. Hold and then release, letting your head drop back to the floor. Repeat this movement thirty times. You should feel your neck muscles flexing and pushing against the palms of your hands.

sagging neck skin. After a few short days of practising this exercise, you should be able to hold your head more upright which will definitely give your posture a boost. You'll look more alert, confident and self-assured.

Tip: Do the Neck Strengthener once a day if you have a thick neck, and twice a day if your neck is long and thin. It's important to remember to use your buttock muscles and the front of the neck when doing this exercise. Many of my clients wrongly use the muscles on the back of the neck, which can result in a neck ache (that's where they get the term, pain in the neck).

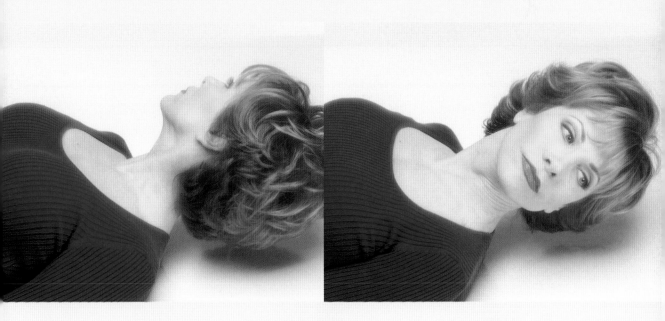

3. Place your arms down by the sides of your body. Keeping your buttocks tight, lift your head and shoulders off the floor a centimetre or so, lifting with the *front* of your neck.

4. Turn your head from side to side twenty times, then relax. Build up to thirty times.

Exercise 11

The Jaw Strengthener

Benefits

This exercise benefits the *pterygoid internus* muscle in the jaw. Working this muscle will help you tone those droopy jowls and will assist in erasing or minimizing the sagging skin along the jawline.

Method

1. This exercise is best done in a sitting position. Assume the basic posture (see p. 51). Open your mouth and roll the lower lip in snugly over the bottom teeth. Pull the corners of the mouth towards the back teeth and roll them in tightly. Keep your upper lip pressed firmly against your teeth. Place your index finger on your chin for light resistance. Open and close your jaw in a slow, scooping motion, using the corners of your mouth to open and close the jaw. Imagine scooping up your favourite ice cream with your 'scoop'.

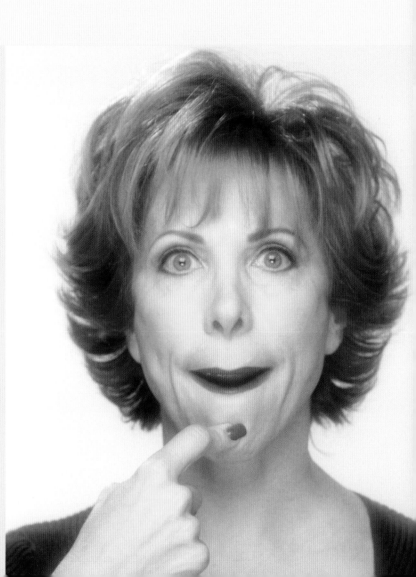

Tip: Make sure you scoop using the corners of your mouth, *not* the jaw hinge. I recommend doing the Jaw Strengthener twice a day to help prevent a sagging jawline. I've also been told by some of my clients that this exercise helps alleviate the painful symptoms of temporomandibular joint syndrome.

2. Pull your chin up about a centimetre (half an inch) each time you scoop. Scoop slowly and concentrate. Visualize the sides of your face lifting. Perform this scooping motion until you can feel the lactic acid burn in your jawline. At this point your head will be tilted back and your chin should be pointing towards the ceiling. Hold your jaw still while visualizing the sides of your face lifting up. Count to thirty while holding this position.

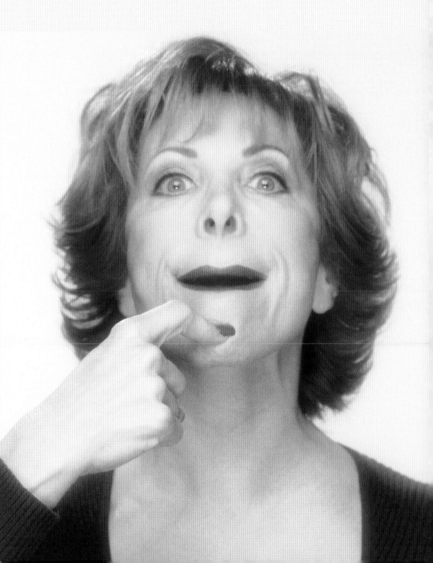

Exercise 12

The Face Widener

Benefits

This is an extremely effective exercise for long, gaunt, narrow faces. It will help widen and soften that gaunt look.

Method

1. This exercise can be done either sitting up or lying down. I like to do this one lying down because I feel I can mentally expand the sides of my face more easily. Assume the basic posture (see p. 51). Open your mouth, pull the corners of your mouth towards your back teeth and roll them in tightly. Keep your upper lip pressed down firmly against the upper teeth. Now visualize big, puffy, fat cheeks coming out of the corners of your mouth. See these fat cheeks filling in the gaunt area. Position your fingertips at the corners of your mouth and make small circular motions on your face. This will mentally help to expand the sides of the face. Continue making these small, circular motions.

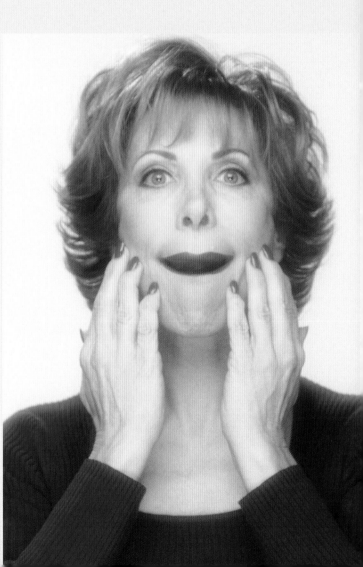

Tip: The Face Widener should be done twice a day to help correct a narrow or gaunt face. If you feel your face is sufficiently wide already, you can definitely skip this exercise.

2. When you begin to feel the muscle widen, slowly pull the hands away from your face while continuing the circular motions. When you begin to feel the lactic acid burn in the sides of your face, make quick circles with your fingers to intensify the energy. Continue this for a count of thirty. Relax and blow between your lips.

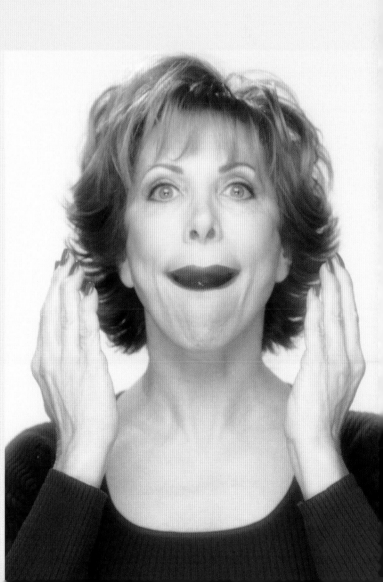

Exercise 13

The Face Slimmer

Benefits

The Face Slimmer narrows, lifts and tones a wide face. If your face is slim already, this exercise will keep the sides of your face toned. Exercising the *buccinator* muscle will increase facial muscle tone. If you're not sure whether your face is wide or narrow, ask a good friend.

Method

1. You can do this exercise sitting up or lying down. Personally, I like to do it lying down because it seems easier, for me anyway, to reverse the pull of gravity from this position. Assume the basic posture (see p. 51). Open your mouth and forcefully roll your lips over your upper and lower teeth. Pull the corners of your mouth in towards your back teeth and roll them in tightly. Place one hand on each side of your jaw, then slowly move your hands up along the sides of your face as you visualize your face lifting. Utilize your mind-muscle connection and visualize the sides of your face moving upwards and outwards, past the jawline, to the top of the head. Look up towards the top of your head with your eyes.

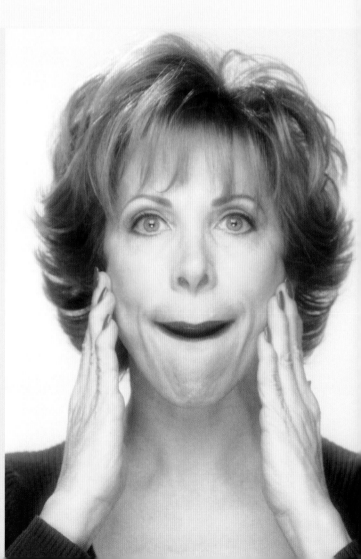

Tip: Do the Face Slimmer twice a day if you have a heavy, full face. If your face is thin, do this exercise once a day for general toning.

2. Continue with this until you feel the lactic acid burn on the sides of your face. When you achieve the burn, keep your hands held above your head, hold that position and count to thirty. Relax and blow out through your lips.

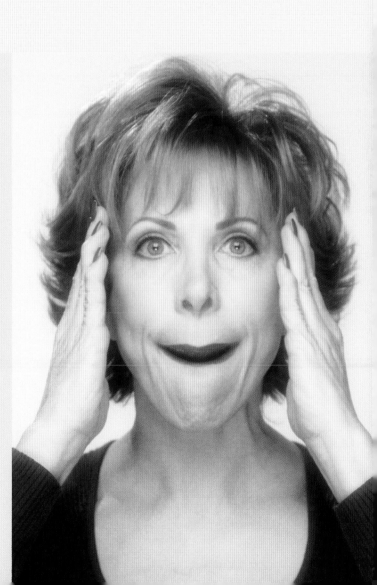

Exercise 14

The Neck and Chin Toner

Benefits

This exercise works and strengthens the *platysma* muscle and is great for firming the chin, neck and jawline. It can greatly reduce double chins and, in some cases, make them almost invisible.

Method

1. Sit tall and straight with your chin held high. Assume the basic posture (see p. 51). Close your lips and smile strongly (a smile without your teeth showing). Place one hand at the base of your throat over your collarbone and pull down slightly on the skin with a firm grip. Look upwards towards the top of your head.

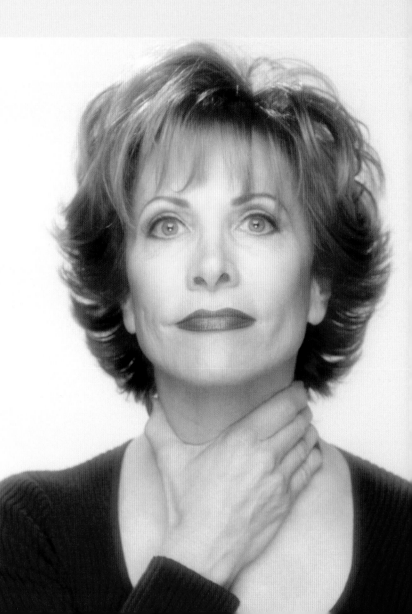

Tip: Do the Neck and Chin Toner twice a day. If you feel you have a double chin problem, do this exercise three times a day.

2. Tilt your head back and release. You should feel a strong pull on the chin and neck muscles. Tilt your head backwards, count to three and return to a normal head position. Repeat thirty-five times.

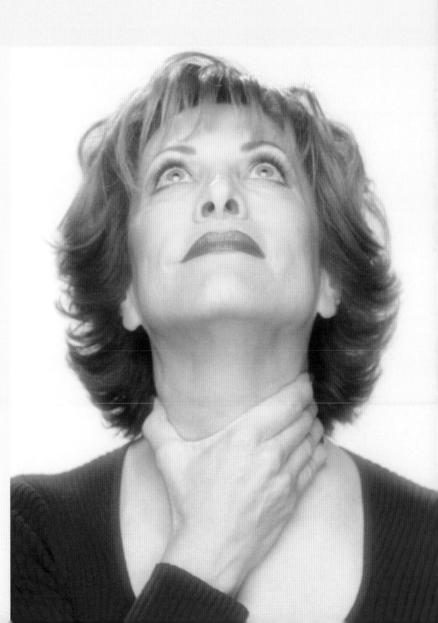

Facercise in the car

Because it's important for you to achieve your goals and because I know most of you have busy schedules, I've adapted all of the exercises so that you can do them in your car while driving to work, to school, to the shops or wherever. These all can be done easily and safely while driving, except the Eye Enhancer, which must only be practised at a red light or while the car is stationary. Be careful and watch traffic lights and other vehicles.

Remember: Do not endanger yourself or others. Take care while you are Facercising in the car even while driving at very low speeds.

Car Exercise 1
Eye Enhancer

Place your middle fingers between your brows and position your index fingers at your outer eye corners. Forcefully squint up with the lower eyelid and feel the outer eye muscle pulse. Now, hold the squint while squeezing your eyes shut tightly. Count to forty. Peek with one eye every few counts to see if your traffic light has changed and continue to squeeze.

Car Exercise 2
Lower Eyelid Strengthener

Place your left thumb at the outer corner of your left eye and your left index finger at the outer corner of your right eye. Squint up and hold the squint, then count to forty while keeping your eyes wide open. Place your thumb and index finger at your inner eye corners. Squint up and then hold for a count of thirty.

Car Exercise 3
Forehead Lift

Place the thumb and index finger of one hand above each brow, in the middle of the forehead and pull your fingers down so that they are above the brows. Push your eyebrows up and release ten times. Then hold the brows up, keeping the fingers pulled down. You'll feel the band of pressure across your forehead. Hold and count to twenty while pushing away on your steering wheel. This movement intensifies the energy.

Car Exercise 4

Cheek Developer

Place the thumb and index finger of one hand on top of each cheek. Open your mouth and pull the upper and lower lips away from each other, thus forming a long, strong, oval shape. Keep the long oval shape of the mouth strong. That's important. Keep the upper lip pressed down firmly against the teeth. Smile with your mouth corners and then release them. Do not use your jaw hinge. Repeat this procedure thirty-five times. You'll feel the cheek muscles move under your fingers. Use your mind–muscle connection and visualize pushing the muscle up under the cheek each time you smile. Push away from the steering wheel each time you smile and release to intensify the energy.

Car Exercise 5

Face Energizer

Pull the upper and lower lips away from each other, which should form a long, strong, oval shape. Use the thumb and index finger of one hand on top of the cheeks. Smile with your mouth corners and release them ten times. You'll feel the cheeks move under the thumb and index fingers. Imagine that you are pushing the muscle up under the cheek each time you smile. On the tenth smile, forcefully pull the upper and lower lips away from each other. Slowly move your thumb and index fingers off your cheeks and up through the roof of the car as you visualize keeping your upper and lower lips pulling strongly away from each other. Count to forty.

Car Exercise 6

Nose Shortener

Use your index finger to push the tip of your nose up and hold it firmly in place. Flex your nose down by pulling your upper lip down over your teeth. Hold this for a second before releasing the lip. Repeat this procedure thirty-five times. You'll feel the nose tip push against the finger each time.

Car Exercise 7

Neck Strengthener

Grasp the front of your neck with one hand as though you were choking yourself. Push your chin away from your body with the front of your neck and towards the windscreen, then relax. Repeat this action thirty times. You should feel your neck muscles flex each time you do this.

Car Exercise 8

Lip Shaper

Press your upper and lower lips together. *Do not* purse them. Be sure not to clench your teeth. Mentally imagine that you are crushing a pencil in the centre of your lips. Place your index finger between the centre of your lips. With the lips pressed together, slowly pull your finger towards the windscreen to lengthen the imaginary pencil. Push against the steering wheel with your other hand. This will intensify the resistance and enhance the exercise. Continue this exercise until you feel a burn in the centre of your lips. Pulse your finger up and down quickly for a count of thirty.

Car Exercise 9

Nasal Labial Smoother

Pull your upper and lower lips away from each other in a long, strong, oval shape. Visualize a line of energy, moving from your mouth corners up to the sides of your nostrils. Use your thumb and index fingers to follow this line upward. Next, visualize that energy beam moving back down that imaginary line toward your mouth corners. Keep repeating this energy movement up and down, using your fingers to follow

and intensify the energy. Do this exercise until you feel the burn, then pulse your fingers up and down for a count of thirty.

Car Exercise 10

Mouth Corner Lift

Press your lips together. *Do not* purse them. Tighten the corners of your mouth into hard knots. Don't clench your teeth. Lightly place your thumb and index finger at the corners of your mouth. Keep sucking in on the corners of your mouth and visualize those corners turning up to make a tiny smile, then turning down to effect a tiny frown. Pull the thumb and index finger away from the corners of the mouth towards the windscreen in small up and down motions to intensify the visualization of your mouth corners at work. Continue with this exercise until you get that lactic acid burn. Hold that burn for a count of thirty, pulsing your thumb and index finger up and down.

Car Exercise 11

Jaw Strengthener

Open your mouth and roll your lower lip in tightly over the lower teeth. Pull the corners of your mouth towards the back teeth and roll them in tightly. Keep your upper lip pressing down firmly against the teeth. Place your index finger on your chin for resistance. Open and close your jaw in a slow, scooping motion. Use the corners of your mouth to effect this, not your jaw hinges. Push away on the steering wheel each time you scoop. Continue scooping until you feel the lactic acid burn. Hold the jaw still as you visualize the sides of your face lifting up. Hold this pose and continue pushing away on the steering wheel while counting to thirty.

Car Exercise 12

Face Widener

Open the mouth and pull the corners of the mouth towards the back teeth and roll them in tightly. Keep the upper lip firmly pressed down against the teeth. Visualize big, fat cheeks coming out of the corners of the mouth. Position your thumb and index finger at the corners of your mouth and make small circular motions on your face. This will help you mentally expand the sides of the face. Continue making the small, circular motions until you begin to feel the muscle widen. When this happens, slowly pull the fingers away from your face while continuing the circular motions and push against the steering wheel for additional intensity. When you begin to feel the lactic acid burn in the sides of your face, make rapid

circles with your fingers to intensify and enhance the energy. Count to thirty.

Car Exercise 13

Face Slimmer

Open your mouth and forcefully roll your lips over your teeth. Pull the corners of your mouth towards the back teeth and roll them in tightly. Now visualize the sides of your face moving up and outward, past the jawline, to the top of the head, pushing away on the steering wheel. Continue moving this mental energy up along the sides of the face until you feel the burn. Hold that position and count to thirty-five.

Car Exercise 14

Neck and Chin Toner

Sit up straight with your chin held up high. Don't get your chin up so high that you disrupt your line of vision, however. Close your lips and smile. Place one hand at the base of your throat, over the collarbone and pull down slightly on the skin. Tilt your head back and release. You'll experience a strong pull on the chin and neck muscles. Tilt your head back and release thirty-five times.

6

Let's get specific

Nine progressive exercises

'VE DEVELOPED A Progressive Facercise programme, consisting of nine facial exercises for people who want more definition or for those who want to develop a specific area of their face.

In the following photos, I've used Gina G., a young lady from California who is a very accomplished actress and singer. I saw Gina perform the lead role of Eva Peron in *Evita* one memorable evening and I was amazed at how she took on the characteristics of Argentina's famous first lady. Backstage, after the show, I asked Gina how she was able to achieve the facial dexterity she showed during the play. She told me that she did my exercise programme and had been doing so for some time. She said she was able to relax and get into character by doing the Face Energizer, the Lip Shaper and the Eye Enhancer. Let's never forget that we all have to 'get into character' if we are going to be successful in our professional and personal lives. Life is one great big stage and there are no dress rehearsals. As Shakespeare said in *As You Like It*, 'All the world's a stage, And all the men and women merely players.'

While the following exercises may, at first glance, seem very much like the basic exercises, there are subtle differences. These exercises work the muscles a little differently to generate more specific and dramatic changes. You may be wondering, why not just do the progressive exercises? Why bother with the basic ones? The answer is simple. You have to learn to walk before you learn to run. You have to build a facial foundation (the essential exercises) before you can move on to the progressive exercises. The essential exercises will work very well for everyone. For someone who wants to fine-tune or correct specific areas, such as hollows under the eyes or fine lines around the lips, then adding the Under-Eye Hollow Lift or the Lip Toner to the basic programme, for example,

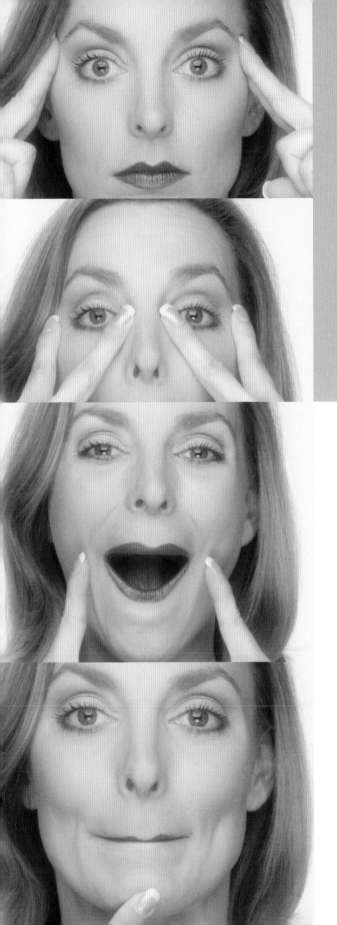

will enhance your progress. Just remember this caveat. Learn the basics first, then progress if you think you need additional exercises for special areas.

Okay. Now let's step it up a notch. We're going to get progressive. When doing these exercises, your posture is important. Before you start you need to suck your navel back towards your spine. Then you wrap (tighten) the front of your thighs towards the back of your thighs and tighten your buttocks. Hold this position as you do the exercise. Before you start an exercise, if it tells you to 'assume the basic posture', this is the position you should be in.

When I say 'press your lips together and blow', I'm referring to the blowing motion necessary to release the lactic acid build-up in the muscles (see p. 51). Remember, even if you don't get a burn on every exercise, still 'press and blow' because it relaxes the face and neck muscles.

Exercise 1

Under-Eye Hollow Lift

Benefits

The Under-Eye Hollow Lift exercises the *orbicularis oculi* muscle which surrounds the entire eye. When the lower eyelid and cheek start to sag, a hollow develops under the eye. This exercise is designed to tone and strengthen the lower eyelids and fill in the hollow.

Method

1. Perform this exercise sitting up. Assume the basic posture (see p. 85). Place your index fingers lightly on the very top of the cheeks and under-eye tissue. Imagine a dot on your upper and lower lip. Open your mouth, pulling these two imaginary dots away from each other to form a long, oval shape. Close your eyes. Roll your eyes to the back of your head.

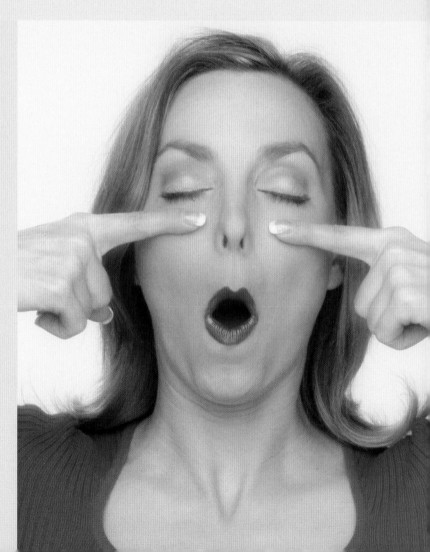

Tip: If you have deep under-eye hollows, perform this exercise three times a day.

2. With your eyes rolled towards the back of your head, open the eyes and quickly flutter the upper eyelids for a count of sixty. You may look like you're flirting but you'll feel a tug at the lower eyelids.

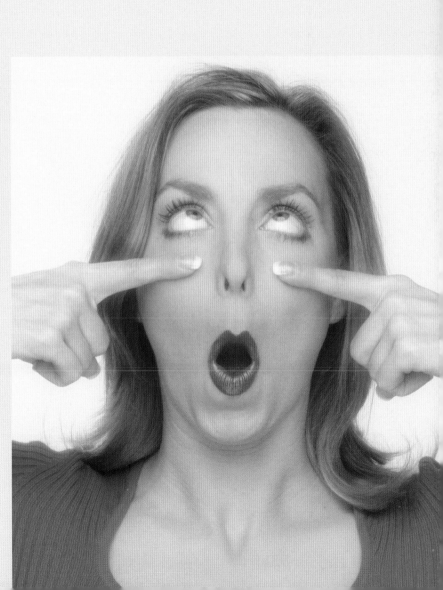

Exercise 2

Eye Opener

Benefits

The Eye Opener helps to maintain the tone of the *orbicularis oculi* and the *levator palpebrae superioris* muscles. When these muscles relax, we get that sleepy-eyed look. We've all seen people like this. They look like they have just awakened or are about to

Method

1. This exercise should be performed sitting up. Assume the basic posture. Place your middle and index fingers at your temples and push up slightly. Focus your eyes straight ahead. Lift your eyelids and relax thirty times, taking care not to arch or raise your eyebrows. Think 'lift and relax' with your upper eyelids.

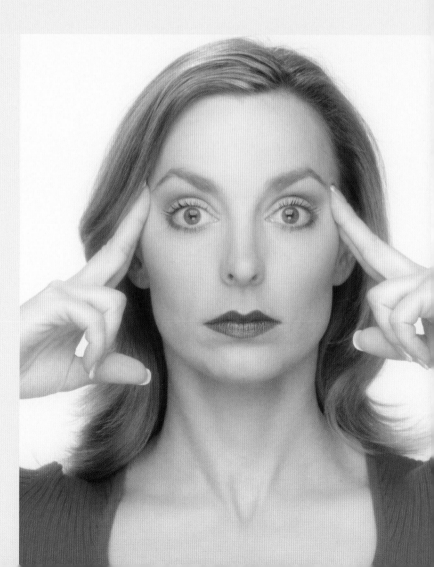

nod off. It's not an energetic look and no one I know wants to look like that. So, this is how we avoid that look. This exercise will keep your eyelids lifted and give your eyes a more open appearance.

Tip: Do this exercise twice daily if you have that sleepy-eyed appearance.

2. Focus your eyes on your knees. Lift your eyelids and release thirty times. Don't arch or raise your eyebrows. Think 'lift and relax' with your upper eyelids. Then press your lips together and blow to release the muscles.

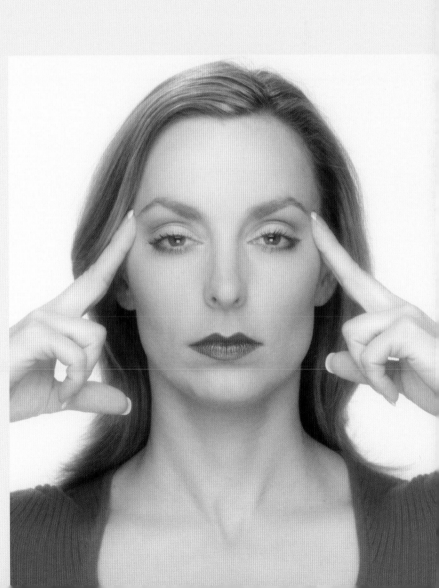

Exercise 3

Cheek Lift

Benefits

The Cheek Lift exercises the *buccinator* muscle. As I've mentioned before, gravity tends to age us by pulling our cheeks down which gives us that flat-faced appearance. We can fight back, however, and here's how we do it. This exercise is designed to lift the cheeks back up where they belong and it helps to add definition to the face.

Method

1. This exercise can be performed in either a sitting position (my favourite) or lying down. Assume the basic posture (see p. 85), but sit with your face forwards and your shoulders back. Imagine a dot on your upper and your lower lips. Open your mouth and pull the dots away from each other and form a long, oval shape with your mouth. Place the index finger of one hand on your chin for light resistance.

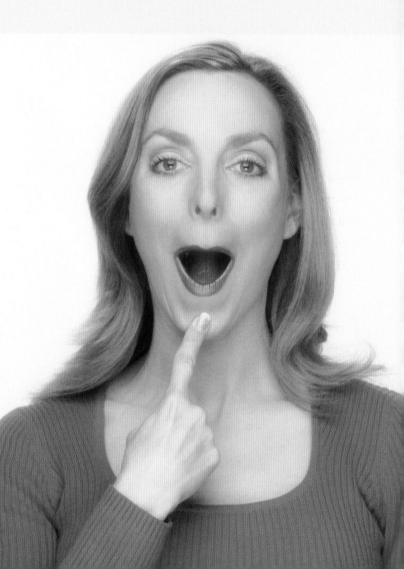

Tip: If your cheeks appear low on your face or you have a flat face, repeat this exercise twice daily.

2. Look up towards the top of your head and squint up with your lower eyelids. Raise your cheeks up by forcing a smile with your upper lip. Push the smile under the cheeks and hold this position for a count of thirty. Then press your lips together and blow.

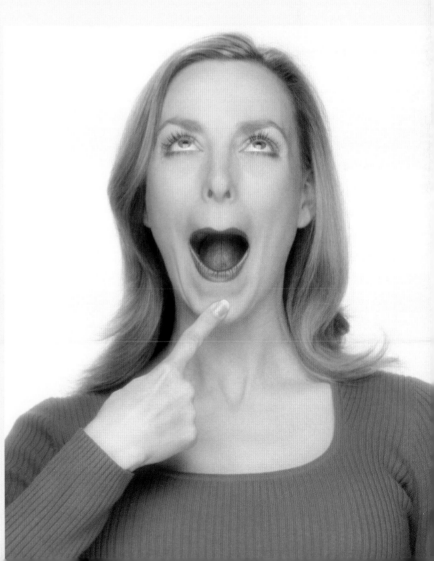

Exercise 4

Lip Toner

Benefits

All major mouth muscles are being exercised with this exercise. Practising regularly helps to enlarge the lips and smooth out lip lines. No more mouths like our mothers'.

Method

This exercise can be performed either sitting up or lying down. Assume the basic posture (see p. 85). Curl your upper lip and pull it in, so that it touches the gums of your upper teeth. Roll your lower lip in towards your lower teeth. Focus your energy in the centre of the lips. Pull down your nostrils. Use your index finger to push the chin muscle up. Concentrate on curling your lips in. Don't clench your teeth. Hold this position until you feel the lactic acid burn and then count to thirty. Press your lips together and blow to relax the muscles.

Tip: To keep the stress lines out of the lips do this exercise twice daily. Alternate between sitting up and lying down to do this exercise.

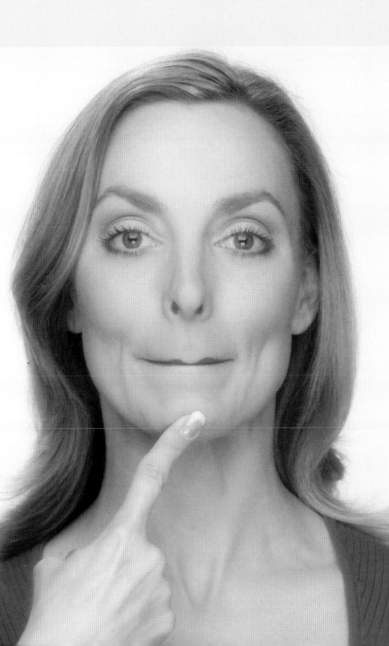

Exercise 5

Lip Corners Up

Benefits

The Lip Corners Up exercise will (guess what?) turn your mouth corners up!

Method

1. This exercise can be done either sitting up or lying down. I like to do this one sitting up because I can exert more mental energy in this position. Assume the basic posture (see p. 85). Open your mouth and imagine a dot on your upper and lower lips. Pull the dots away from each other so that your mouth forms an oval shape. Keep this oval shape by pressing your upper lip against your teeth, then smile with your mouth corners quickly eighty times.

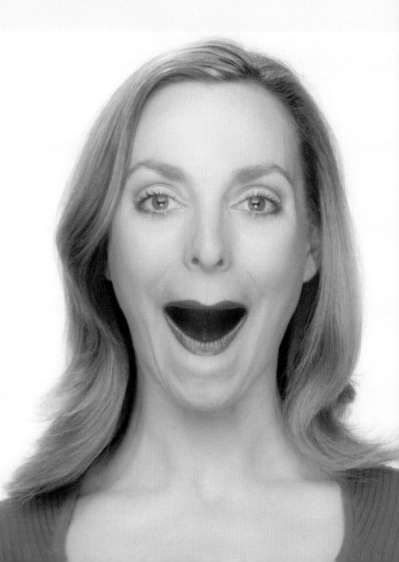

Tip: Do this exercise twice a day and be prepared to see a very quick, positive change in your lip corners.

2. You'll feel a burn in the mouth corners. When this occurs, pulse your index fingers (see p. 51) at the corners of your mouth for a count of thirty. Press your lips together and blow.

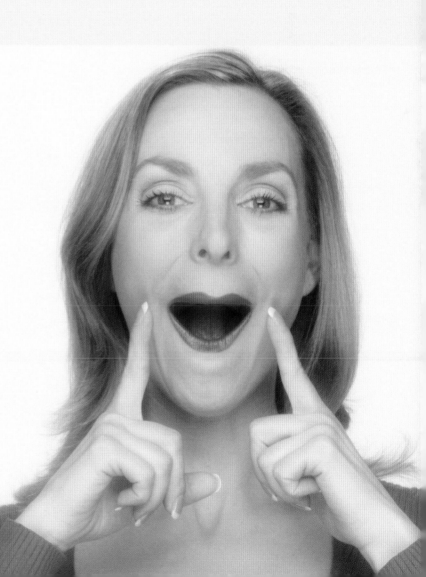

Exercise 6

Lower Face Lift

Benefits

The Lower Face Lift works and tones the major muscles of the jaw and the mouth. It helps to firm up the jaw area and improve the frame of your face.

Method

1. Do this exercise sitting up. Assume the basic posture (see p. 85). Open your mouth wide and roll your lips over your teeth. Pull the corners of the mouth towards the back teeth and roll in tightly. Look up towards the top of your head and smile so your mouth corners are pointing towards the tops of your ears.

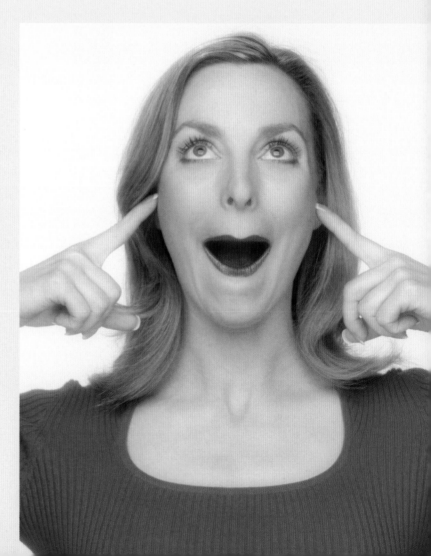

Tip: This exercise is great for firming the lower face. Do this exercise twice daily to strengthen and tone this area.

2. Place the index fingers at the corners of the mouth and draw an imaginary smile line (think happy face) with your fingers from your mouth corners towards the tops of your ears. Hold your fingers above your ears. Push your face forward and throw your shoulders back. Go for the burn and count to thirty. Press your lips together and blow.

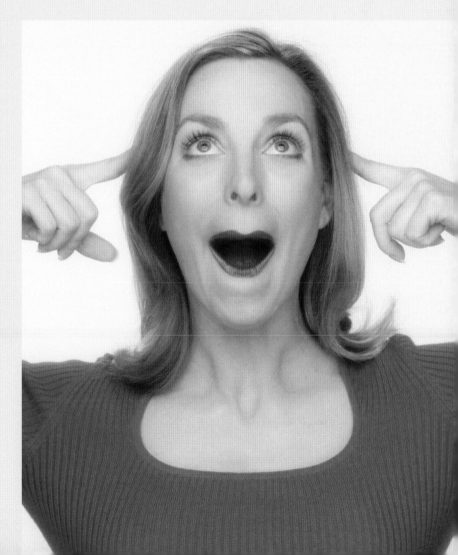

Exercise 7

Lower Eyelid Firmer

Benefits

This Lower Eyelid Firmer strengthens the *orbicularis oculi* muscle around the eyes and firms up the lower eyelids. The effects of this exercise will be diminished under-eye hollows and more muscle in the upper cheeks.

Method

1. Perform this exercise sitting up. Assume the basic posture (see p. 85). Place your middle fingers at your inner eye corners and your index fingers at your outer eye corners. Pull your upper and lower lips away from each other, so your mouth forms a long oval shape.

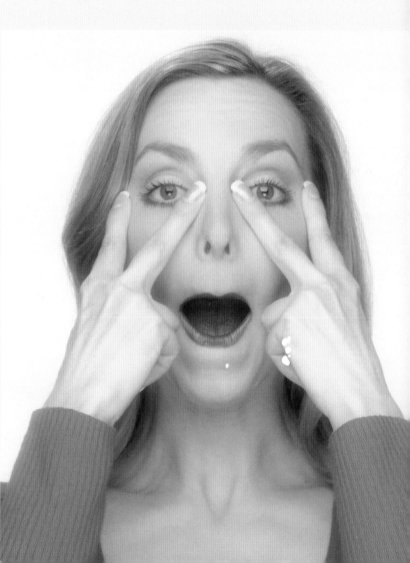

Tip: This is a great exercise for those of you who have excessive under-eye hollows or under-eye puffiness. If you fall into this category, repeat this exercise twice daily.

2. Keep your upper lip pressed down against your teeth. Squint up strongly with your lower eyelids and smile with your mouth corners, pushing the energy up under the cheeks. Look up at the ceiling and hold this position for a count of ten. Release and repeat this exercise four times.

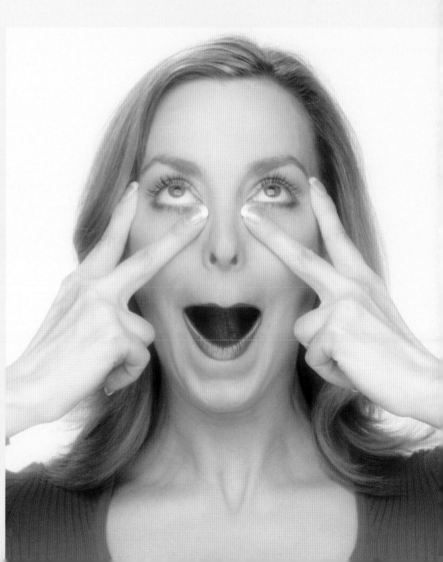

Exercise 8

Defined Face Energizer

Benefits

The Face Energizer in the previous chapter and the Defined Face Energizer may seem similar, and they are. However, this more advanced exercise will fill in the flat area between the sides of the nose and the cheeks, which the Face Energizer is not designed to

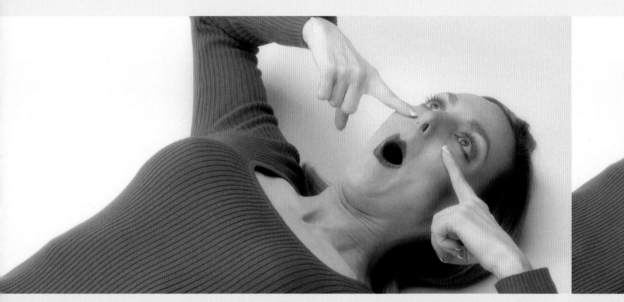

Method

1. Perform this exercise lying down and assume the basic posture (see p. 85). Imagine a dot in the middle of your upper lip. Now imagine a dot in the middle of your lower lip. Open your mouth and pull these two imaginary dots apart to form an oval shape with your mouth. Place your index fingers lightly on the top part of your cheeks. Smile with your mouth corners and release, feeling the cheeks move under your index fingers. Visualize the muscle pushing up under the cheek each time you smile. Repeat the movement ten times.

do. This action adds softness to the face and makes it appear more youthful. The exercise works the *orbicularis oris* and the *levator labii superioris* muscles to build up this area.

Tip: To add more definition, perform this exercise twice daily.

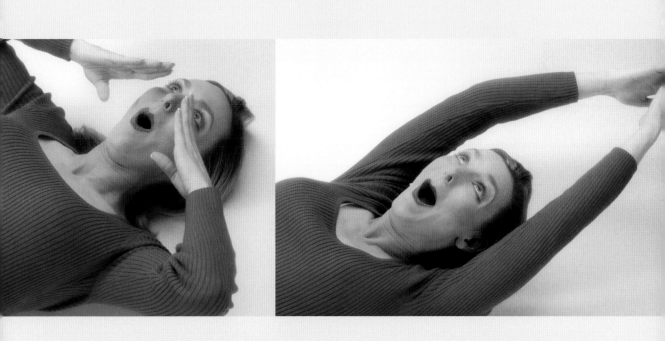

2. On the tenth smile, utilize all of your strength to pull the upper and lower lips away from each other. Imagine that your cheeks are moving along the sides of your nose, through the middle of the eyebrows and up through the top of your head. Lift your hands off your cheeks and follow the energy along the sides of your nose, through the centre of the eyebrows and on through the top of your head. Hold this position for a count of thirty.

3. Lift your head about a centimetre (half an inch) off the floor or so, using the muscles in the front of your neck and your tightened buttocks. Keep your hands above your head and hold the energy for a count of thirty. Press your lips together and blow to relax the muscles.

Exercise 9

Lip Line Smoother

Benefits

This exercise smooths the lines in the upper lip.

Method

1. Perform this exercise in a sitting position and assume the basic posture (see p. 85). Imagine a dot on your upper and lower lips. Pull the dots away to form a long, oval shape with your mouth. Roll your lips over your teeth. Look up towards the top of your head. Place your middle finger in the centre of your upper lip and place your index finger and your ring finger on either side of your lip and apply pressure.

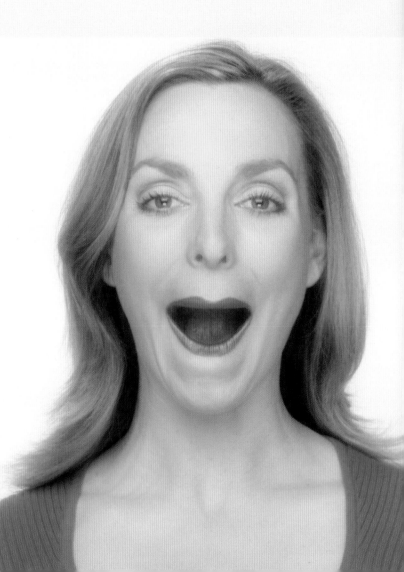

Tip: Keep pressing down on your lips with your fingers. This exercise is fabulous for smoothing out the upper lip lines.

2. Hold the long 'O' with your mouth and smile with your upper lip quickly forty times. Hold the smile and imagine your upper lip is pushing up to your nose. Hold this for a count of twenty. Press and blow.

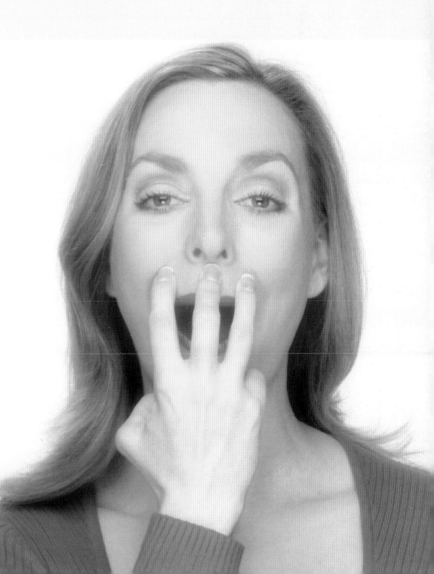

7

Skincare essentials

I BELIEVE IN A natural, consistent and disciplined approach to looking and feeling good. Whether we talk about a beauty or an age-control regime (both preventative and corrective) this approach is essential if we are to retain both inner and outer youth and beauty. To paraphrase W. Somerset Maugham, 'Youth and beauty are ecstasies, the same as hunger.' As well as exercising the muscles of the face and body, there are many health and beauty aids that can have a dramatic impact on what the mirror reflects back. We know that Facercise is going to help us achieve a youthful appearance but there are other factors to be considered in our quest for the ever-youthful face we all want and can have. Everyone wants to know the secret to staying young. Lucille Ball once said, 'The secret of staying young is to live honestly, eat slowly and lie about your age.' That's one way of looking at it. But I'm going to teach you a better way: the Facercise way to staying youthful.

Skin specifics

The skin is amazing. To start with it's the human body's largest organ, it protects the other organs very efficiently, wards off infections and toxins on a twenty-four-hour basis and performs a myriad of other amazing feats. It comprises about fifteen per cent of our total body weight. The approximate chemical composition of the skin is as follows: water 70 per cent, protein 25.5 per cent, lipids 2 per cent, trace minerals 0.5 per cent and everything else 2 per cent.

The skin is comprised of three main layers: the epidermis, the dermis and the subcutaneous tissue. The epidermis is the thin, outermost layer of skin and consists of three interwoven types of cells – keratinocytes, which produce the protein, keratin; melanocytes, which produce the sun-tanning pigment called melanin that protects us from the harmful ultraviolet radiation of the sun; and the Langerhans cells, which intercept foreign substances that attempt to pass through the skin.

The epidermis is the primary site of skin cell growth. New cells push mature cells upwards. When these mature cells reach the top layer of the epidermis (the *stratum corneum*), they die and flake off. New cells appear on the epidermis every twenty-eight days or so, but this cycle can be accelerated by conditions such as sunburn, harsh cleansers and skin irritations. The epidermis can be nourished through careful skin cleansing and moisturizing.

The dermis is the middle layer of the skin. It forms about ninety per cent of the skin's thickness. This complex layer of skin contains a tight and sturdy mesh of collagen and elastin fibres. Collagen is responsible for the structural support and elastin contributes to the skin's resiliency. The dermis also contains the sebaceous glands (sweat glands), hair follicles and a small number of nerve and muscle cells. Sebaceous glands, located around the hair follicles, produce sebum (an oily protective substance that lubricates and waterproofs the skin and hair). When the sebaceous glands produce inadequate amounts of sebum, the skin dries out and becomes more susceptible to wrinkles. Overproduction by the sebaceous glands often leads to the formation of blackheads and pimples, also known as acne. The sweat glands secrete water and salts. The oil and water created in the dermis form an emulsion that protects and lubricates the epidermis. This emulsion helps prevent oil and moisture loss, which in turn helps normalize the acid (pH) balance of

the skin. The condition of the dermis decisively shapes skin tones and contours.

The subcutaneous tissue is the innermost layer of the skin. This tissue is found under the dermis and consists mainly of fat. The function of the subcutaneous tissue is to act as a 'shock absorber'. It gives the skin its flexibility and resiliency, insulating the body and protecting underlying tissues from injury. This tissue also functions as a storage site as it absorbs chemicals, drugs and nutrients. The loss of this type of tissue often occurs with age and leads to facial sags and more pronounced wrinkles.

Most of us are born with normal skin, but genetics and lifestyle choices can compromise our skin's well-being (and our overall well-being) as we age. You can improve the health and vitality of your skin by improving your personal habits. Start with a dedicated skincare programme, a diet rich in fruit, vegetables and fibre, face and body exercising, appropriate protection from the elements, adequate amounts of sleep and constructive stress management. Making appropriate and consistent lifestyle choices is the key to looking and feeling good.

The skin is shaped by bone structure and underlying muscle tissues. It is also moulded by the protein-based connective tissues in the dermis, which contain collagen and elastin. Collagen and elastin are the skin proteins responsible for elasticity, tone and texture. Collagen forms the structural network of our skin. It provides the skin with the strength and durability required to protect us throughout our lives. Elastin also assists in maintaining skin resiliency and elasticity. As we age, collagen and elastin start to diminish, leading to signs of ageing such as thinning skin, wrinkles and facial sagging. Full bee-stung lips, which have been injected with collagen, are seen on many movie stars now and are definitely in vogue. But they are very costly and painful and they are also temporary. Since collagen and elastin can never be naturally restored to ageing skin, all exercise and especially facial exercises can help compensate for this loss of these essential elements by building up the underlying muscles, which will greatly improve the strength and beauty of your skin.

I've divided my top skincare tips into six sections

- Skin protection
- Nutrition and supplements
- Exercise and deep breathing
- Sleep and stress management
- Skincare basics
- Skincare secrets

Skin protection

A good, daily preventative skincare regime is paramount if you want to maintain a healthy, glowing, youthful complexion. It is *essential* even at a young age because today's poor lifestyle choices inexorably lead to tomorrow's skin disasters. Your skin is an external organ and most of it is exposed to the outside elements all of your life. It's no wonder that it ages faster than any other organ of the body.

The skin is highly susceptible to many things, but the worst element it ever encounters is the sun. The sun supercharges the normal ageing process (intrinsic ageing) dramatically. It thickens the skin on a permanent basis. This process is called photoageing and needs to be taken very seriously to avoid skin tumours and deadly skin cancers. A tan looks great but it's probably the most unhealthy thing you can do to your skin. I am always amazed when I hear people tell me they are going into a tanning booth to get a mega-dose of artificial sun. That's really like going to a place where they cook things (a kitchen with a big oven, maybe) and having yourself cooked a little bit every day. A tan is really the result of the body trying to protect itself against burning. The body knows that a tan isn't good for it. It doesn't want to get cooked, even a little bit. If you look at areas of your body which have not been exposed to the sun (your buttocks, for instance), you'll notice that the skin in that area is not dry, rough or discoloured. Smooth as a baby's bottom, so the saying goes. Lack of ultraviolet exposure to these areas leaves the skin clear, smooth and light. Lack of any extensive exposure to the long ultraviolet rays of the sun means that these dangerous rays have not penetrated into the layers of your skin. It's this intrusive penetration that causes the cosmetic ravages we call ageing. The rays of the sun also unleash molecular mutants called free radicals, which are discussed at length on p. 110. The sun's ultraviolet rays also wreak havoc on the proteins that would normally keep your skin smooth, flexible and strong. This carnage results in all the things we associate with ageing: dry, wrinkled, sagging, uneven skin, discoloration and an excellent chance of developing some type of skin disorder, which could include skin cancer. Here are some excellent ways to protect yourself from the sun:

- Avoid the most harmful rays of the sun. Stay in the shade from 10am until at least 3pm.
- *Always* wear a protective layer of at least SPF 30 sunscreen to ward off ultraviolet radiation.
- *Always* protect your face with a wide-brimmed hat and wear polarized sunglasses designed to protect your eyes from the harmful ultraviolet radiation.

Nutrition and supplements

Your skin is a reflection of your lifestyle and choices. What you put into your body dramatically influences your skin colouring and texture and it can also affect how you feel. Okay, so what should we be putting into our bodies? For starters, we need:

Water and other beverages Water is a fundamental part of our lives. It's the universal solvent, aiding in digestion and absorption of food. It also ferries nutrients and oxygen to every cell in the body while flushing out toxins and other wastes that accumulate. Drinking at least eight glasses of water a day has been a mantra for many years, and for good reason. Drinking this amount of water will keep your skin clear and assist in keeping your muscles toned and healthy.

Low water intake is known to be one of the main culprits in speeding up the ageing of the skin. Many people think that if they drink soft drinks, tea, coffee, beer or other alcoholic beverages, that they don't need to drink lots of water in addition. These beverages, however, do not take the place of water, because the body processes them differently.

Along with its many other benefits, water also aids in weight loss. Since it contains no calories, water can serve as an effective appetite suppressant and it assists the body in metabolizing stored fat. Studies have shown that if you are overweight according to average height and weight comparison charts, you should drink one glass of water, in addition to the recommended eight daily glasses, for every eleven kilos (twenty-five pounds) you carry over your recommended weight.

If you aren't drinking enough water, your body will start to retain water to compensate for what it knows is a water shortage. To eliminate fluid retention, drink more water, not less. Some people say bottled mineral water contains fewer toxins than tap water and is healthier for you. You literally are what you drink.

Alcohol is another major culprit when it comes to water retention. It's very high in empty calories, creates puffiness in your face and body and dehydrates the skin. You need to drink at least one full glass of water for every alcoholic beverage you consume. Water can help your body to metabolize and excrete the alcohol more efficiently. How much alcohol is too much? Well, some people drink to steady their nerves. When they get so steady they can't move – that's too much.

A healthy diet

Totie Fields once said, 'I've been on a diet for two weeks and all I lost is two weeks.' I love that saying. How many of you have been on a diet where you didn't lose anything, especially your appetite? Someone once referred to her type of diet as being 'a seafood diet'. 'I see food and I eat it.' Well, that may work for some people, but it's not recommended if you want beautiful skin. We need to remember that healthy nutrition is an integral part of the Facercise programme. Eating an unhealthy diet, such as one high in fat, salt or sugary foods, will not give us the nutrients to build muscle effectively nor will it enable us to generate the energy and enthusiasm that is necessary if we are going to change our facial contours. If your goal is to build strong, supportive facial muscles and also to gain a fabulous clear complexion while you seriously slow down the ageing process, you need to become aware of nutrition and supplements. Good nutrition provides the body with the essential nutrients and elements it needs daily, such as vitamins, minerals and protein.

Nutrition is a highly personal matter. The diet and supplements that work for one person may not be appropriate for another person. An excellent way to learn which kinds of minerals your body (and skin) need is to have a nutritionist draw a blood sample and send it to a laboratory for a detailed analysis. Your food intake and supplement programme must fit your individual needs, which depend on your age, the state of your health, your lifestyle, body type – even your psychological profile. You need to ask yourself if you are hyperactive and nervous, or placid and easy-going. Are you a positive person who sees the glass as half full or a negative person who sees it as half-empty? Or do you just see a big glass with nothing in it? You have to be able to identify yourself before you can start to work on yourself. These attitudes can make major differences in your nutritional requirements.

Unless you've recently arrived here from another planet, you've most probably been exposed to more different diets than Carter has liver pills. You've probably tried the no-fat diet, the no-carbohydrate diet, the meat-free diet, the no-sugar diet and maybe even the no-food diet. There's probably even a diet called the 'you-can-eat-anything-you-want-as-long-as-you-don't-swallow diet'. You name it. It's been tried. Hopefully, you've absorbed some modicum of nutritional wisdom along the way and since this is such a personal thing, whether it's the Atkins diet or the Jenny Craig diet or something in between, if it works for you, then do it. There is no diet that works for everybody. My advice is to eat until you explode. Boy, can you lose weight that way. Just kidding! My serious advice is to eat a variety of different foods. Make sure you eat the right amount to achieve a healthy weight. If you're not sure what an optimum, healthy weight would be for you, consult your doctor.

You should eat one to two portions of good-quality protein each day. Choose lean beef, chicken, turkey, fish or eggs. Protein is needed for growth and repair of the connective tissues within the skin. Vegetables and fruits high in fibre are always a safe choice for a healthy lifestyle, so try to eat five portions a day. The vitamins and minerals in fresh fruits and veggies are great for feeding your skin and for assisting your body in building and repairing cells. Many nutritional studies support the findings that vitamins C, E and A, plus minerals such as selenium and zinc, help to combat the breakdown of collagen and elastin, the skin's supporting and connective tissues.

It is best to avoid foods that contain saturated fats or sugars, whenever you can. Sugar has been called a woman's instant upper. But remember. What goes up must come down. And coming down from a sugar high can be a rough, bumpy ride. Eating foods high in sugar content is a sure-fire way to gain weight because sugar brings empty calories into the equation – lots and lots of them. We're not sure whether sugar intake causes acne, but it does wreak havoc with your complexion, making it appear drawn and dull.

You should also exercise caution when seasoning food with salt. Salt creates water retention so that your face and body look puffy. Try to remember that the two main ingredients in salt (sodium and chloride) are deadly by themselves. They neutralize each other when they come together to form salt. Keep that in mind when you have the salt shaker in your hand. Substitute herbs and spices in place of salt for flavouring, whenever possible. You get enough salt in your daily diet to satisfy your body's requirements without adding one single shake of salt to your food.

Anti-ageing supplements

I believe that everyone needs to understand the theory proposed in 1954 by Dr Denham Harmon, which is almost universally accepted by the medical community today. Dr Harmon's theory goes directly to the heart of the ageing process that occurs in every human being. He stated that the body contains free radicals. These unfriendly little atoms or groups of atoms are created, in part, by the way our cells utilize oxygen to produce energy. Free radicals are unstable oxygen molecules created during the body's basic metabolic functions, such as digestion and breathing. All these little guys have one thing in common: they contain at least one unpaired electron. This creates a problem. If an electron is unpaired, another molecule or atom can hook up with it. This 'bonding' creates a chemical reaction which may not always be positive. Picture someone hooking up with someone else after a few drinks at a cocktail party. Maybe it's a right match. Maybe not. So, what does all this scientific information have to do with ageing, you ask? It has *everything* to do with ageing. Free radicals don't have a long lifespan – maybe just a split second – but that's enough time for

them to do some serious damage to neighbouring cells when these 'bondings' are mismatched. These unholy alliances can cause reactions which, it is speculated, contribute to heart-muscle-cell damage, nerve-cell damage, cancer, hardening of the arteries, and a host of other health-related degenerative disorders which may number as many as eighty at the time of writing this. Dr Harmon's studies ironically pointed out one of life's great paradoxes. Most free radicals are oxygen-based. We need oxygen to sustain life, yet oxygen promotes free radicals, which cause ageing and disease.

It should be pointed out that not all free radicals are harmful. In fact some are definitely beneficial because they help destroy viruses and bacteria which attack our bodies. They also help to produce some very necessary hormones and enzymes which are vital to human life. *Most* free radicals are *not* beneficial to us, however, and we need to do all we can to avoid overwhelming our body with these hostile invaders.

It's bad enough that our own bodies manufacture free radicals, but it gets worse. Air pollution, radiation and sunlight, not to mention cigarette smoke, all create free radicals. If you smoke, or associate with people who smoke, for example, you need to be aware of the horrendously toxic elements in cigarette smoke. Remember, these toxic elements contribute to the proliferation of free radicals.

We can also stimulate the proliferation of free radicals by being out in the sun. When we are out in the sun, unprotected, even for a very short period of time, molecules in the skin absorb the sunlight. Once these molecules are activated, they turn into free radicals almost immediately. They then turn on their neighbour molecules as described above. Free radicals attack and injure vital cell structures such as collagen and cellular membranes. These attacks eventually leave small defects in the skin, which eventually turn into wrinkles. Again, I cannot stress this enough: stay out of the sun and avoid cigarette smoke whenever possible.

It's important to note here that Dr Harman was the first to expound the free radical problem, but another doctor named Imre Nagy expanded on Dr Harman's theory. Dr Nagy agreed with Dr Harman that free radicals were the primary causes of ageing and age-related problems, but he went a step further. He suggested that most of the ageing damage was experienced by the outer layers of the cell. Prior to Dr Nagy's theory, most scientists and dermatologists believed that primary free radical damage was experienced by the interior of the cell, causing cellular DNA damage and, hence, ageing. But Dr Nagy was able to prove that DNA extracted from the cells of older humans, even those past ninety years old, was able to reproduce normally. Since the DNA was not damaged, DNA damage couldn't be the primary cause of ageing. From the findings culminating from Dr Nagy's research, scientists have been able to develop antioxidants which are designed to penetrate cell membranes, aid in the repair of these cells and increase their ability to retain water, which is vital to the cell's well-being. (Without water, the cell becomes dehydrated.) The work of these two doctors, among others, has proven invaluable in the development of treatments which can probably help reverse the signs of ageing.

What can we do once the damage is done? This is a good question. Fortunately, there are certain nutrients known as antioxidants, which have proven extremely effective in slowing down or even reversing the ravages of the free radical assault on our bodies. Antioxidants are compounds which aid the body in disarming the free radicals, so to speak. They are instrumental in helping our bodies deactivate or at least minimize the free radical ravages within our cells. These antioxidant warriors can prevent free radicals from running amok in the body by giving these mutant molecules new electrons to replace the ones they've lost. Once the antioxidant hooks up with the free radical, the free radical is stabilized and ceases its pilfering activity against neighbour cells. The antioxidant actually neutralizes the free radical and renders it harmless. They can also help repair sun-related damage caused by free radicals and they may even help reduce the risk of skin cancers. So what are antioxidants? They are vitamins, minerals and other substances found in a variety of common foods. Here is a list of some of the top antioxidants:

■ **Selenium** Top foods containing selenium include seafood, meat, Brazil nuts, tuna, wholegrains, cottage cheese and chicken. As well as having antioxidant properties, selenium also seems to help relieve anxiety: in one university college study most of the men and women who took a daily dose of 100mcg of selenium for just five weeks reported feeling less anxious, less depressed and less tired.

■ **Betacarotene** Orange and dark-green vegetables, such as spinach, carrots and sweet potatoes, are rich sources of betacarotene. High levels of this antioxidant seem to cut the risk of lung, mouth, throat, oesophagus, larynx, stomach, breast and bladder cancer.

■ **Vitamin C** This can be found in all fruit and vegetables but particularly good sources are citrus fruits, broccoli, green and red peppers and strawberries. The Nobel Prize-winning scientist Linus Pauling, who lived to be ninety-three, stated that we could add twelve to eighteen more years to our lives by taking 3,200 to 12,000mg of vitamin C a day.

■ **Vitamin E** Nuts and seeds, including peanuts, almonds, sunflower and sesame seeds, and wheatgerm are all rich in vitamin E. Dr Eric Rimm, author of a Harvard study on the role of vitamin E in the prevention of heart disease, said, 'The risk of *not* taking vitamin E is equivalent to the risk of smoking.'

■ **Other antioxidants** Vitamin B12, vitamin A, folic acid and pycnogenol are also beneficial antioxidants. Pycnogenol, which is an extract of pine bark, is considered to be the most powerful antioxidant available at the time of writing this, and it has proven extremely effective against environmental toxins. Research indicates that pycnogenol is twenty times stronger than vitamin C. Pycnogenol activates vitamin C and gets it working hard before it leaves your body.

Caution: Because everyone's biochemistry is unique, it would be prudent for you to consult with a nutritionist before embarking on any antioxidant supplement programme. It goes without saying that no pregnant woman should take any vitamin, mineral or food supplement without first consulting her doctor.

Exercise and deep breathing

From the moment we're born, we must breathe in oxygen to survive. Apart from being essential for the production of energy, oxygen is vital for synthesizing fats, proteins, carbohydrates and other substances in food, thereby helping to build and maintain cells, organs, muscles, bones and other structures.

The most effective way to clear your skin, through increased oxygen intake, is to exercise at least three times a week. Exercise makes you look and feel better. After a good workout, your skin will take on a healthy glow. Aerobic exercise increases blood circulation which, in turn, enhances the flow of oxygen and nutrients to your skin. Clinical studies conducted in various countries throughout the world have proven that regular aerobic exercise (elevating the heart and breathing rates for thirty minutes or more, at least three times a week) keeps you healthy and fit. It's also a tremendous stress buster. If you're not that athletic, even mild exercise such as a thirty-minute brisk, daily walk, will help get your blood pumping and your complexion glowing.

Physical activity greatly benefits the skin by increasing the flow of blood throughout skin tissue and introduces oxygen and other nutrients needed for the maintenance and repair of the skin cells. Oxygenated blood helps dispose of toxins and internal pollutants, which can damage skin and connective tissues. When you exercise to the point where you make your skin flush, you can see the colour change in your skin. This is the oxygenated blood, coursing vigorously throughout your body, replenishing as it goes.

Caution: If you are over forty or have not exercised recently, you should seek the approval of your doctor before initiating any kind of exercise programme.

Exercise and deep breathing

Deep breathing is a mild (but effective) form of aerobic exercise. Like Facercise, it can be done anywhere. You can do it while driving, sitting at your desk, while you're in a lift or doing the housework. Deep breathing will make your heartbeat speed up, pumping more oxygenated blood throughout your body. Like an internal massage, deep yogic breathing will give you a calm, energized feeling.

Most of the time we take short, shallow breaths, utilizing only the upper portion of our lungs. Deep breathing means breathing from your diaphragm located in your stomach area. You literally have to teach yourself the art of deep breathing. Here's how you do it. Sit up straight with your shoulders relaxed. Do not lean forward. Inhale through your nose. Slowly fill your lungs with a deep breath. Try to expand your lower ribcage as you inhale. Eventually, you should feel the air moving into the top of your lungs. When you've reached maximum breathing capacity (when it feels like you're going to pop), hold your breath for ten full seconds. Then slowly exhale through your mouth. Relax and breathe normally for four breaths. Repeat this procedure ten times. Deep breathing is a helpful and effective way to elevate your energy and clear your skin.

Sleep and stress management

Sleep is absolutely vital for human beings to survive. Everyone knows that sleep is good for a person and we all know how revitalized and refreshed we feel after a good night's sleep. What many people *don't* know is how sleep refreshes and nourishes the skin. I call lack of sleep a beauty bandit, as it robs us of the essential rest and recuperation our skin needs to look its best throughout our lives. When you don't get enough sleep, your face will pay for it. Your reward for skipping your sleep is a tired, droopy face. When our system begins to shut down, we need sleep. Without it, muscles become fatigued and the face will begin to droop and sag, or worse, take on a sallow, dull appearance. Then other problems start to develop. The blood pressure and the pulse begin to drop. This results in less blood and oxygen being pumped to the facial area. In short, you aren't going to be looking too good. People are going to think you need to get some sleep, and they're right. International studies indicate that an alarming number of people are sleep-deprived. Everyone should get at least seven to eight hours of sleep a night to look, feel and be your best.

We go through different stages as we sleep. We start out in a light sleep (the *theta* state). Then we enter the *delta* state, when we are in deep sleep. This is when your body is regenerating. Tension and the problems of the previous day are reduced to a minimum during this time. The deep sleep period doesn't last all that long, however. Within an hour or so, you enter another state, known as the Rapid Eye Movement (REM) stage. During this stage, your brain is functioning almost as though you are awake, but you're not. Your body remains asleep. Your mind is back at work, however, resolving problems, releasing thoughts, etc. We go through several stages of REM activity and this is good. The more REM sleep a person gets, the more likely it is that they will wake up feeling refreshed, energized and positive. During a normal seven to eight hour sleep span, you will probably have four or five REM sleep episodes. The last REM episodes last the longest and are the most beneficial, which is why getting seven to eight hours of sleep a night is so critical. Some people think they need less than seven hours' sleep. Not true. Others don't get the necessary hours because of lack of physical exercise, poor eating habits, consumption of alcohol or caffeine or disturbances during the night. Anyone who says they can get by on less than seven to eight hours of sleep a night probably looks the worse for it.

Skincare basics

There are three main types of skin: normal, oily and dry. Most people have a combination of these types of skin, for example normal skin with an oily panel in the centre. You need to remember that, as skin starts to age, it also starts to deteriorate, and so your skincare routine needs to be modified accordingly. For instance, as we age, the amount of secretion the oil glands produce can decline and I've had people tell me their skin is changing because it's less oily now than it used to be. I tell them the reason this is happening and tell them they do not want to lose any more moisture in their skin by using harsh cleansers to wash away the oil, or astringents to reduce the amount of oil.

Normal skin

Normal skin has it all: good muscle tone, resiliency and optimum hydration. Normal skin appears soft, plump, moist and has a healthy colour. It literally glows. If you have this skin type, you should cleanse it both in the morning and in the evening, and use protective moisturizers, as well as a sunscreen with a minimum SPF rating of thirty during the day. At night you should apply hydrating creams to rejuvenate tired skin before bedtime.

Oily skin

Oily skin is usually hereditary and is the result of overactive sebaceous glands. It often can be recognized from its thick, shiny and somewhat slack appearance. An oily skin sometimes will appear to be dirty or neglected. The pores of the skin will probably appear to be enlarged, due to oil that is trapped in the pilosebaceous follicles. There may be a few blemishes on the chin or forehead areas and the skin will feel oily to the touch.

Heat and humidity complicate oily skin problems. A person who has oily skin and lives in a place where it's hot or humid will most probably find their skin is even more oily. Using harsh soaps, or making excessive use of astringents or scrubs can make oily skin worse. The use of exfoliating products, such as enzymes and botanical products, can help regulate the oil and improve the look and texture of oily skin.

If you have this type of skin you must pay special attention to thorough (but gentle) cleansing morning and evening. Protective moisturizers containing humectants (substances that attract and hold water) will assist the skin in maintaining the suppleness and moisture it requires. I often have clients who will tell me that they don't think they need to use a moisturizer because, they say, 'I have oily skin.' I tell them that even though their skin may be oily, they still need water because normal skin contains both of these elements. And don't forget the sunscreen. A common misconception among people with oily skin is that they don't need a sunscreen. Wrong. And make sure it's a sunscreen with a minimum SPF rating of thirty.

Dry skin

In people with dry skin, the sebaceous glands are underactive – they do not produce enough of the secretions required to properly moisturize the skin. Dry skin is also a by-product of the ageing process. The body's activity slows down as we grow older and the oil gland activity slows down as well. Dry skin, lacking the necessary oil content, is unable to retain moisture, since oil in the skin acts as a natural barrier to moisture loss. The characteristics of dry skin include fine, delicate, thin skin with tiny, superficial lines. This type of skin wrinkles easily.

Problems with dry skin are intensified by exposure to the sun and improper skincare. Proper care for dry skin should include daytime and night-time protection, using rich moisturizers and sunscreen with a minimum SPF rating of thirty. Proper cleansing is also a must, but only once a day, preferably right before bedtime. Excessive cleansing will strip away whatever natural oils are in the skin and further dehydrate the skin, exacerbating the dry skin problem. Use rich, creamy face cleansers to clean and soften the skin.

Skincare secrets

Following are some techniques for a healthier skin and tips on buying the best skincare products.

Dry brushing

This is a technique that hails from Baden Baden, one of Europe's oldest and most renowned beauty spas. It is the most effective way I know to detox and nourish the skin on my body. Before taking a bath or a shower, use a loofah mitt made from dried sisal. Massage your body, using a circular motion, starting at the bottom of your feet and working up your body. Use a loofah strap to shimmy up the back of your body, starting with the ankles and working up to the shoulders. Rinse the strap and mitt once a week and let them dry overnight.

By stimulating blood circulation and sloughing off dead skin cells, this daily treatment energizes you, revitalizes the lymph system and also assists in eliminating toxins from the skin. Dry exfoliation promotes a healthy, pink glow and soft, smooth, fresh-feeling skin. An additional benefit is that it is cost effective to the extent that it will save you the expense of body lotion, which you will not need if you perform this procedure daily. A good-quality sisal loofah mitt should last you a year or so.

Exfoliation

No skincare regime is complete without exfoliation (the clearing away of dead skin). Regular exfoliation with a botanically based enzyme mask will get rid of the old skin cells and bring in the new. Enzymes fall within a classification of proteins known as dynamic proteins. These temporarily attach themselves to molecules in the skin. In doing so, the molecule becomes ionized, transformed into a positively or negatively charged particle. Enzyme skin tighteners are protein enzymes which will enter the skin and hydrolyze the dead tissue. When enzymes are rinsed and removed, the dead tissue will flood out of the skin. In my experience, the enzyme masks that work the best contain protein, RNA, L-lysine and proline. These cleanse and penetrate the skin to tighten the epidermis. A good enzyme mask will constrict, tone and tighten the skin while drawing out impurities from the pores.

Avoiding night-time wrinkles

One of the most common complaints I receive, on a daily basis it seems, is about what I like to call the 'wrinkles on the face when I wake up' syndrome. Some people are truly horrified when they glance in a mirror upon wakening. This is because many people sleep with their face in the pillow. They don't start off sleeping that way, but because of night-time tossing and turning, they end up face down in the pillow when they wake up. Most people don't think they move around that much during sleep, but studies have shown that many people gyrate quite a bit during a night's sleep, as they move from *theta* to REM sleep and back again.

You can't control your dreams but you can control your position when you sleep. A good habit to initiate is to sleep without a pillow under your head. While this may seem uncomfortable at first, it is the best way to get a good night's sleep without moving around all that much. You can use a neck roll, if you feel you need something but put that pillow under your knees and lie flat on your back when you fall asleep. This will definitely cut down on your nocturnal gyrations and will result in a sound, healthy, beneficial good night's sleep. And you won't wake up with a 'pillow face'.

When we dream, we move our faces. We frown, smile, grimace, etc, just as we do during the day. To reduce the lines in the forehead or between the eyebrows, you can apply surgical tape on the skin furrows before going to bed. You may not look all that attractive, but you have some decisions to make here. Do you want to look good when you're asleep or when you're awake? Tough decision, right? Not really. When you discover that your skin looks smoother in the morning, you'll know which way you want to fly. I routinely tape the area between my eyebrows before I retire every evening because I like the way I look when I wake up.

Transdermal and oxygen-based products

The products I have found to be most valuable in aiding the skin are *transdermal* (i.e. they penetrate the skin). This allows the product to store in the skin for a period of time, so that it can favourably influence the functions of cells and glands located within the dermis. Your best bet for locating high-quality transdermal products is to talk to your dermatologist or a licensed esthetician.

Some cosmetic manufacturers claim that *oxygen-bearing* emulsions can actually penetrate the skin and bring other nutrients such as vitamins A and B directly into skin cells to perform repair work. Do you recall me saying that oxygen is the great vehicle for producing energy and continuous rejuvenation of our bodies? Oxygen-bearing cosmetics are some of the most highly touted products in today's cosmetic markets. The main active ingredient in oxygen cosmetics is medical-grade hydrogen peroxide. Bacteria, which contribute to skin problems such as acne, cannot survive in an oxygen-rich environment. This would seem to indicate that oxygen acts as an anti-bacterial agent whether on or in the skin.

One oxygen-based cosmetic I often use happens to be hydrogen peroxide solution (3 percent). Pour a bottle of hydrogen peroxide solution into a plastic spray bottle. Spritz it on your face in the morning and you will look and feel refreshed. I pour a little bottle of solution in my bath after a long day and I feel as though I've had a total body facial. A hydrogen peroxide solution bath is also a great remedy for jet lag. But be careful – full-strength hydrogen peroxide is bleach.

The latest products

Recently I was in a fine department store, looking at the latest batch of 'miracle creams' and other products on prominent display. As usual, my curiosity got the better of me and I began reading what some of these things do for your face. One immediately caught my eye. It came in a beautiful coloured jar and as I was reading the contents, a saleslady came up to me and started telling me about all the miraculous things the cream could do for my face. It contained a patented copper peptide complex, I was told, and it had been tested on burn victims, severe acne sufferers and various other unfortunates. 'If it can heal damaged skin and replenish the collagen in those people,' she gushed, 'imagine what it can do for you.' I didn't buy the product but I left the store thinking to myself, 'How is the average person ever going to be able to tell what is hype and what is real?' The truth is, skincare is a mega-big business now. New formula items appear hourly, it seems. And it's lucrative. Anti-ageing skincare products grew in sales by twenty-five per cent from 1999 to 2000 and are, at the time of this writing, the fastest growing segment of the cosmetic business. How do you know if it works or not? It's *caveat emptor*, according to Dr Richard Glogau, a San Francisco dermatologist. Let the buyer beware. With this in mind, the following names will increasingly be on the products you buy. Here is an explanation, though some may already be familiar to you.

■ **Alpha Hydroxy and Beta Hydroxy** – Available in prescription and non-prescription strengths, these acids remove dead skin cells, revealing newer, tauter skin.

■ **Copper Peptide** – Supposedly aids rejuvenation of the skin and reduction of wrinkles.

■ **Fullerenes** – Water-soluble fullerenes (carbon spheres shaped like a football) show intriguing potential for skincare. Much smaller than liposomes and nanosomes, they are building blocks for collagen, incredible carriers for skincare ingredients and, most importantly, they show promise to become potent free radical scavengers.

■ **Furfuryladenine** – This is an anti-withering agent found in the leaves of green plants. Early studies indicate that it might help reduce signs of sun damage such as blotches, fine wrinkles and roughness of the skin.

■ **Heavy Water** – Deuterium Oxide (D20) is a rare water found in a few saline lakes and in deep seawater. It feels and tastes like regular water but it is ten per cent heavier, hence the name. Being heavier helps it to resist evaporation and it dries out more slowly, which is what makes it so useful in skincare products.

■ **Retinols** – These are vitamin A derivatives and are available in prescription and non-prescription strengths. They are supposed to build collagen and regenerate the elastin which allows skin to stretch.

■ **Spin Traps** – Just when it seemed as though free radicals were gaining the upper hand in the battle to age us all as fast as possible, scientists have discovered a new substance which allows them to assemble an A-Team to turn the tide in the battle against ageing. These new team members, called spin traps, are intelligent anti-oxidants. They are nitrone-based substances which trap free radicals and examine them to determine how to most effectively prevent them from causing skin cell damage. They also appear to possess anti-inflammatory properties, which would make them a tremendous weapon against the factors that age skin. Spin traps have enormous potential for helping skin stay healthy.

Sun damage

Even though scientists continue to help prevent ageing with wonderful new substances, it's always going to be paramount to remember what I have been stressing throughout this book. *Most of the signs of ageing are the result of sun damage.* You simply *have* to stay out of the sun. If you are going to be outside, at least stay in the shade during peak sun hours and wear SPF Factor thirty sunscreen, even in the shade. Says Dr Norman Levine, a University of Arizona dermatologist, 'All the stuff that is sold in the drug stores pales in comparison to the use of sunscreens for the prevention of wrinkles.'

8

A final word

A MIND IS a terrible thing to waste. So is a face. And your mind is all that really stands between you and the face you deserve. Reflect on this for a moment. Visualize your life style, your eating habits, your exercise (or lack of it) and all the other things you do over the course of a busy day. All of these things affect the way you look. And, since we all really do care about how we look (if we're honest with ourselves), why not make a few beneficial changes in areas where these changes will enhance your looks, benefiting you in the long run?

Every exercise I have outlined, every tip I have discussed, has been designed to benefit your skin and your face. I pamper my skin every day of my life because I am not going to be able to trade it in later for a newer, younger model. We have to play the hand we've been dealt, but we have options on which cards we keep and which ones we throw away. This is what Facercise is all about. The techniques I have placed before you in this book will teach you how to play the game successfully and end up with a winning hand.

In the many, many years I've been advocating and teaching Facercise, I've met many hundreds of thousands of people from all walks of life, throughout the world. I've watched them undergo truly remarkable, even miraculous, changes in their faces and their lives by incorporating Facercise into their daily life patterns. Eleven minutes a day, twice a day is not a large chunk of time out of anyone's daily routine. And small investments, prudently made, can yield spectacular dividends. After all, $5000 dollars invested in Microsoft or Dell Computers in 1990 was worth millions and millions of dollars ten years later. Was that 'small' investment worth it? You be the judge.

Facercise has taken me on a truly remarkable journey around the world. It's a far cry from my skincare clinic in Monterey, California, all those years ago. I've loved every minute of the journey, which continues on, for me anyway, for ever. I used a quote in my first book, which is a favourite of mine. It's an old Chinese saying which states, 'When the student is ready, the Master appears.' There are students all over

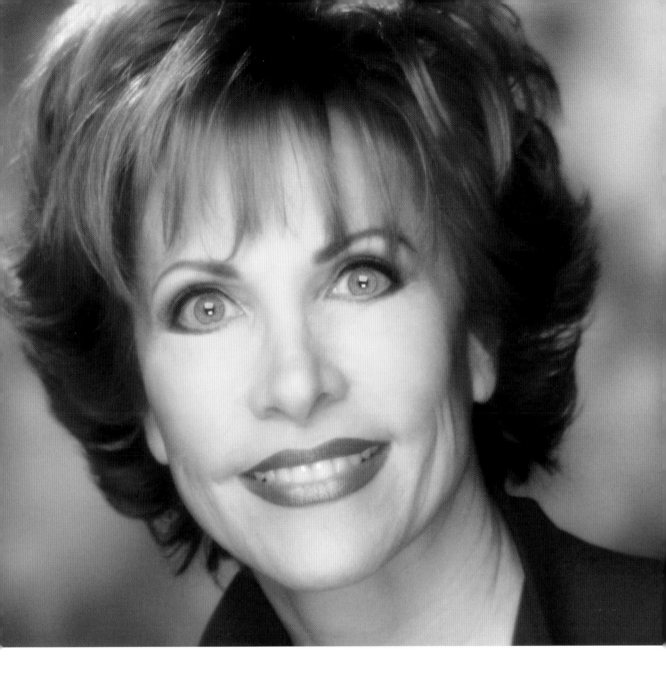

the world who are ready now and Facercise is ready for them. It's never too late to do something truly beneficial for you and your face. It's your face. Make the most of it.

Whenever you need encouragement, revisit the 'before' and 'after' photos of the ladies pictured in the book. Those dramatic photos should give you all the encouragement you need to stick with the programme. If you need more motivation, read some of the testimonials I've reprinted from the thousands and thousands of letters I've received over the years from satisfied clients worldwide. Facercise changed their lives for ever. It definitely changed mine. It can do the same for you.

Testimonials

These are some comments from clients who have used Facercise to enhance and improve their lives and their looks. I hope their words will encourage you to persevere.

Dear Carole,

Thank you so much for putting your time and energy into developing Facercise. Where would I be without it? Like many of your clients, I've undergone cosmetic/reconstructive surgery – three major operations – to correct considerable damage caused by a head-on collision with a drunk driver.

I don't handle anaesthesia very well and I needed two additional operations. The information I got from Facercise eliminated the need for additional surgery by correcting the problems to my satisfaction (and I'm rather picky). Thank you again.

Annie Bess
Los Angeles, CA

Dear Carole,

I was born with a hemangioma on the left side of my face, which grew rapidly. To slow the growth until I was strong enough for surgery, the doctor placed eight radioactive seeds around the growth. We assumed the seeds were gone along with the growth. Then, last year, I began to experience pain and numbness in my face. Seven doctors later, they discovered the seeds, still there, still radioactive,

killing my skin and building up layer after layer of scar tissue. I suffered quite a bit of muscle and nerve damage. Then I discovered your book.

Your exercises did what six weeks of physical therapy couldn't. Now the numbness is almost completely gone and I noticed a definite improvement in the muscle tone. I am so thankful I discovered your book. I have recommended Facercise to my friends and I even told my surgeon how helpful it was to my recovery, since he had asked me what I was doing to improve the damage so quickly.

Sincerely,
Lisa M.
Omaha, Nebraska

Dear Carole,

I first borrowed your book from the library. I must say that I had my doubts about it. After starting the exercises, I decided to buy the book. I'm very enthusiastic about it. Facercise can not only change the shape of your face but also the shape of your mind. I've always been self-conscious because I felt my face was too thin and long. I was able to widen my face and give it a shorter appearance as well as enlarge my lips and build up my cheeks. At thirty years old, it was hard to believe I could make such dramatic changes.

Many thanks,
Biruta van Demer
The Netherlands

Dear Carole,
I read about your beauty regime in *Harpers & Queen* – the one where they called your techniques one of the top one hundred beauty tips in the world. That seemed to be a rather tall claim, but I decided to give it a try. I am truly amazed at what I have been able to accomplish in a short period of time. You've not only perfected one of the top beauty programmes in the world; you've succeeded in turning back the hands of time. My congratulations to you and my thanks, also.

MaryAnne Thornton
London, England

Dear Carole,
I live in Australia and have been in the sun for many years. When I saw you on TV, though, you looked very well and you said that you had spent a lot of time in the sun when you were young and I thought to myself that your exercises could work for me. I purchased your book and it's been the best investment I have ever made. I notice a lot less fine lines in my face now and my skin seems much smoother now. Thank you so much for all the information you have chosen to pass along to all of us who need it.

Anne Randall
Melbourne, Australia

Dear Carole,
I was afflicted with Bell's palsy. I picked up your book at the suggestion of my physician. I started doing your exercises and I was relieved of numbness almost right away. My eye, cheek and mouth corners have all turned up back to normal. I think it's a miracle and I want to thank you from the bottom of my heart for your book and your help.

Yours happily,
Jennifer Wharton
Abbotsford, BC

Dear Carole,
It's hard to believe that in an ocean of frauds and 'me-too' book authors that there really is an island of authenticity in you and your programme. I was badly injured in an accident and have had numerous surgeries to correct the damage. If it weren't for a seriously compelling desire to avoid additional surgery, I would have given up after the umpteenth person promised me visible results with their facial exercise programmes. When someone like you

shows up and you really can produce the goods, it almost seems too good to be true and skepticism results. It isn't easy separating the chaff from the wheat. Your programme sure did, though.

You have probably been told this a million times, but you are a very special and dynamic lady and your Facercise programme is just fantastic.

Sincerely,
Katie W.
Studio City, California

Dear Ms Maggio,

My jaw had a serious problem and the left side of my face didn't move well and became weak. I was afraid of being seen by other people and didn't want to go out at any time. I tried your wonderful book and I'm now much better and I'm no longer afraid of going out. I have regained my confidence and I don't know what I would have done without your book. I really would like to say thank you, Ms Maggio.

Thank you truly,
Seiko Inouye
Tokyo, Japan

Dear Carole,

I have been doing your exercise programme now for about ten months and I can't believe the difference I made in my face with just that little bit of exercise I was doing, working my facial muscles. Not only did my facial looks improve, but quite frankly, the highest motivator for me is the release of tension. I noticed a big improvement with TMJ (sore jaw joints) and neck problems I was having from tension.

With sincere thanks,
Sara Bengston
Denver, Colorado

Dear Carole,

I wanted to write and tell you that I was getting facial toning treatments with the Galvanic Pulses once every week. If I didn't go every week, my face would start to fall. At thirty years old, I felt totally dependent on these treatments. I saw you when you were on Dateline and literally ran out to buy your book. I started the exercises and stopped the toning treatments. Not only did Facercise work, but it worked better than my toning treatments and it only cost me $12.95. What a bargain.

Thank you so much for giving my self-esteem a much-needed boost.

Love,
Joannie Davis
New York, New York

Dear Carole,

I have wanted to write you a thank you letter for some time now, so here it is. When I first found out about Facercise, it was in August of 1998. At that time I had weaned my son and was experiencing postpartum depression. Also, I had lost the last ten pounds that I was holding on to from the pregnancy, all at once. You see, once I lost those last ten pounds, my face literally dropped. I became even more depressed. I went to see a dermatologist who advised me to try a chemical peel or perhaps, at a later date, the laser. After that visit, I found your book in my local health food store. Well, that day my life took a new turn for the better. You see, before Facercise, I'd actually dodge mirrors in my own home. Now I can look at my own reflection and smile. I was able to widen my face, make my cheeks higher and fuller and tone my jawline, just like you promised in your book.

Much love and peace,
April Besch
Brightwater, New York

Carole,

I wanted to drop you a line to thank you from the bottom of my heart for your wisdom and expertise. You probably don't remember me, but I came up to you after one of your seminars in London to discuss my double chin and wide face. You were kind enough to give me some pointers and spend a few minutes talking to me even though you had other people in line to see you. I have been doing the neck toner exercise, as you suggested, and just yesterday, one of my oldest friends asked me if I had undergone surgery or liposuction to lose my double chin and narrow my face. I should have told her yes. Instead, I gave away my secret and told her about your book and your video. When *Harpers & Queen* magazine named your programme as one of the top one hundred beauty products in the world, it should have been number one. Thank you. Thank you. Thank you.

Dilys Hampton
London, England

Dear Ms Maggio,

I've been an actor and have noticed that doing Facercise greatly helps my facial expressiveness. You never mentioned this in your book but I think it's something that would be sought after by performers, even if they didn't need the anti-ageing aspect. Your face becomes more alive and you can project better.

Thank you again,
Denise Michaels
New York, New York

About the author

CAROLE MAGGIO is a licensed esthetician who has gained wide-ranging attention in the international media. Facercise, developed by Ms Maggio over twenty years ago, is a widely accepted alternative to cosmetic surgery and has been used for years by celebrities, rock stars, royalty, business leaders, and politicians. Ms Maggio is also a bestselling author who has spent decades researching facial exercise techniques and passing them along to her countless thousands of clients worldwide. She currently lives in Redondo Beach, California.

Facercise was recently voted one of the top one hundred beauty treatments in the world by *Harpers & Queen* magazine and Ms Maggio has been called the world's foremost authority on facial exercises.

For information about Ms Maggio's video and audio tapes, private classes, seminars, her world-renowed skincare line or any of her beauty products, you can call 800-597-3555 or 310-540-8048. Her fax number is 310-540-0581.

You can also visit the Facercise web site at facercise.com or you can e-mail Carole at: cmaggio@mminternet.com

Ms Maggio's postal address is:
Carole Maggio Facercise, Inc.
409 N. Pacific Coast Highway #555
Redondo Beach, Ca. 90277
USA

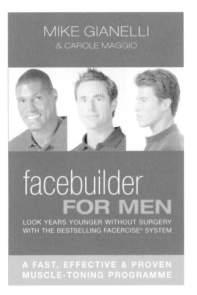

Also by Carole Maggio and Mike Gianelli

Facebuilder for Men

In *Facebuilder for Men* Carole Maggio turns her attention to her largest-growing market. Using the principles of bodybuilding – isolating and working the muscles one by one – she shows how to develop and tone your facial muscles, tighten your skin and improve your complexion. With these scientifically designed, precision exercises you can firm and define a sagging jawline, smooth facial lines, reshape your nose and reduce under-eye puffiness.

Devised specially for men, the exercises are simple, easy to follow, and illustrated with black and white photographs. They can be performed anywhere – even in the car.

Follow *Facebuilder for Men* and you can dramatically improve your appearance in only six days.

Available now from Pan Books
0 330 49030 3
£6.99

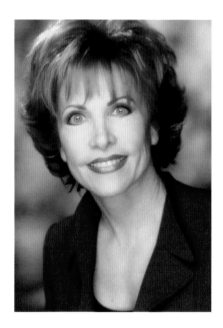